Wade through all the misinformation and ...

Be Healthy, Be Happy

Your Personal Trainer's Assistant

Ron Fay, P.E.

with **Barbara Fay, RN, BSN**
AFAA Certified Personal Trainer

NV Home Base
I enjoyed exercising
with you!
Barb Fay

Fay's Fitness Company

Fay's Fitness Company
41 Owego Road
Candor, NY 13743
www.faysfitness.com

ISBN 0-9706920-2-1

Authors: Ron and Barb Fay
Illustrations: Dale Fay
With contributions by Rebekah Fay

Printed by
First Capital Graphics
315 North George Street
York, PA 17403

This book is dedicated to those that struggle to reach their fitness goals, yet do not employ the services of a personal trainer. Your struggle will be difficult, as time will be wasted, safety will be compromised, and your motivation will wane. Our thoughts are with you.

Other books by Ron Fay and Fay's Fitness Company:

Small Club Start-up – A Personal Trainer's Guide
A guide for personal trainers on how to start their own small fitness club. Based on the author's experience of opening and running a club since the mid 1980's. Helps those considering starting a club avoid all the pitfalls.

Keeping on Track Training Journal—An affordable fitness journal designed for personal trainers to distribute to their clients. Contains 12 weeks of daily nutrition and exercise diary sheets.

Table of Contents

Guy Gullible

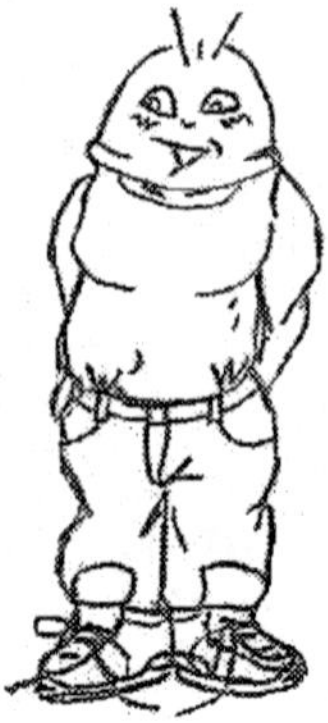

Lisa Stickbody

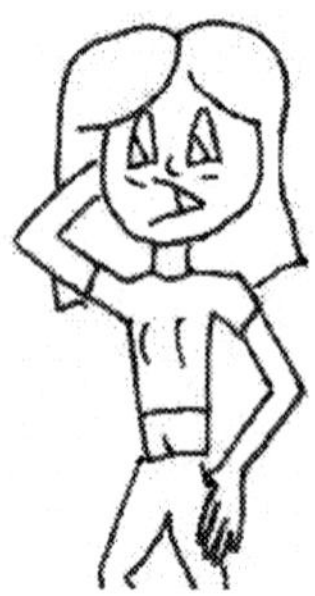

Jim Trainer

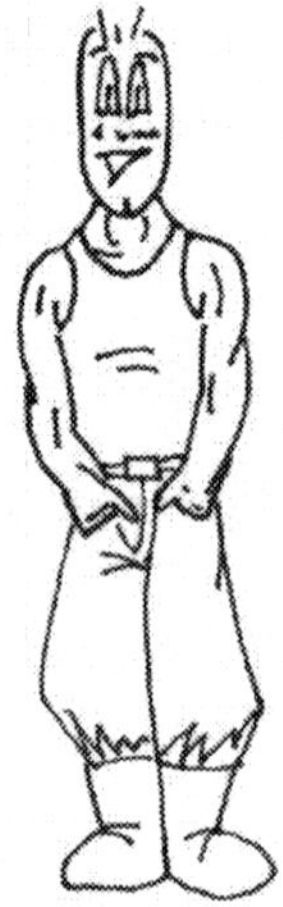

Jill Trainer

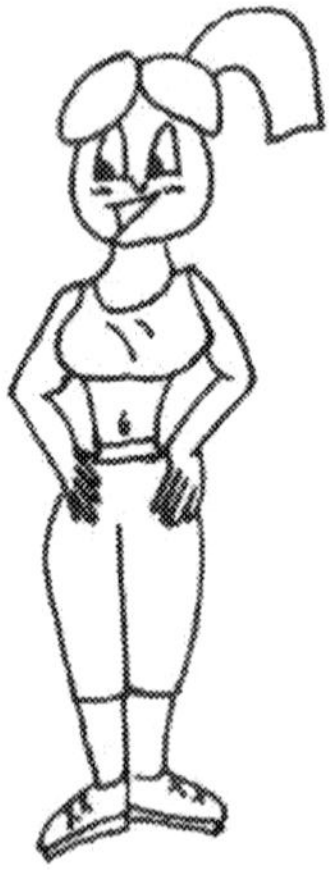

Joe Knowitall

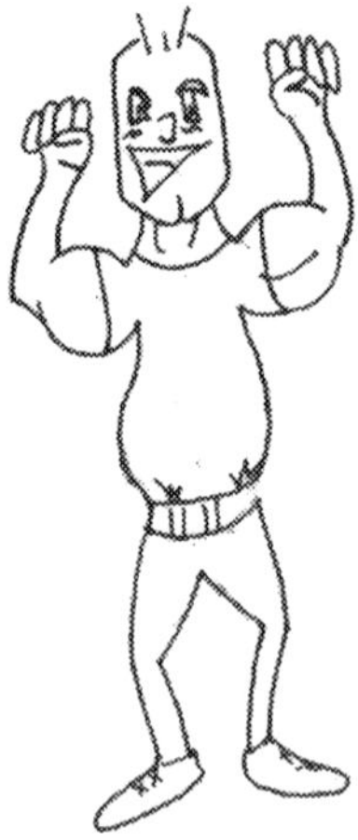

Jim Trainer and Friends

By Dale Fay

Foreword

Why should I hire a personal trainer?

It is possible that you *wouldn't* benefit from hiring a trainer. If you are in great shape; have no difficulty getting motivated; do continual research of and practice the safest, most effective forms of exercise; and can look objectively at your exercise program to determine what works and what doesn't; then you really don't need a personal trainer.

The rest of us would benefit.

We need to face up to the fact that the majority of us are not active enough to get in shape and that we desperately need help. 61% of Americans are overweight and only about 10% of us exercise regularly.

By nature, we constantly look for ways of getting out of activity. We park as close as we can to the store entrances. Machines do all our physical work in the home. Automobiles take us everywhere so we don't have to walk or ride our bikes. We are so conditioned to do the least amount of physical work possible, that when it comes to exercise, it seems contrary to our nature. We put so much effort into getting out of doing physical work, exercising for the sake of staying fit is difficult - in fact it's down right hard work! If you haven't exercised in a while, Newton's Law - a body at rest will stay at rest until acted upon – will work against you when you decide to get up and going.

Consider this scenario: At your annual check-up, your doctor informs you that you need to exercise. Perhaps he mentions that the 20 extra pounds you are carrying around gives you increased risk for diabetes, heart disease, hypertension, cancer, etc. So you pay for an annual gym membership, but only go for the first few weeks. Or maybe you go out and walk regularly for a while. Before you know it, you're back at the doctor's office again listening to him telling you should exercise. Newton's Law at work.

You have an alternative. Break the cycle. Hire a trainer.

Consider these benefits of hiring a personal trainer:

Motivation: Trainers help coach you through your workouts. They hold you accountable and give you the extra push you need to stick with a program.

Knowledge: A good trainer knows the safest, most effective way to help you meet your goals. They will have an objective view of your fitness program and will save you time exercising by getting efficient results.

Record Keeping: A trainer will track your progress toward your goal and get you where you want to be efficiently.

Even those of us that have regular exercise routines can benefit from using a trainer. They are experts in the best and safest way of achieving fitness goals. They can help you modify your program to make it more effective.

But they're so expensive!

The main obstacle to overcome for many people is paying a trainer. "They're so expensive! Some trainer's get $100 per hour! How can I afford this?"

Here's an idea: trade in your automobile for a bicycle and then you'll have plenty of money to work with. In fact, you'll get plenty of exercise riding to work as well. After all it's your health!

Seriously, the main consideration should be becoming healthier and developing a program that works. A trainer should eventually work herself out of a job. The plan is to get you educated and to overcome the 'body at rest' thing. Once you are knowledgeable of what works for you and you are moving, then the trainer has done her job. Now

Newton's other law – a body in motion stays in motion – can take effect.

As far as what trainers are compensated, most are grossly underpaid. Let's consider an average trainer charging $50 per one-hour training session. Keep in mind most trainers can do no more than 20 sessions per week. The times they are not training they are recruiting, traveling, promoting, or designing programs. They have to pay for their own health insurance, (subtract about $500/month X 12 months = $6000) and vacations (2 weeks), so in this case, the trainer would have a gross yearly income of about $44,000. This does not take into account expenses! Chances are, they are working many more hours than the 40 hours per week and making the same amount of money.

How do I find a good trainer?

Here are some things to look for:

- Someone you like and trust. This person will be your friend and confidant. You will be telling her all about yourself.
- Knowledgeable. You'll want a safe and effective work-out. If your trainer quotes "no pain, no gain" to you, find another one.
- Proven record for getting results. You should start seeing results within 4 weeks of working with the trainer. The trainer should be recording these results for you and show you how you are making progress.
- Prompt and courteous. You need a trainer that will keep appointments and will stay in touch.

A note about certification: Your trainer should be certified with a major training organization, but more important than this, are the above points. Focus on hiring a trainer you like and trust; one that will get you where you want to be, safely.

The particular certification the trainer has should be secondary, keeping in mind that being certified typically means they have taken a course with the certifying organization, have passed written and practical exams, have required CPR training, and need to get continuing education credits to maintain it.

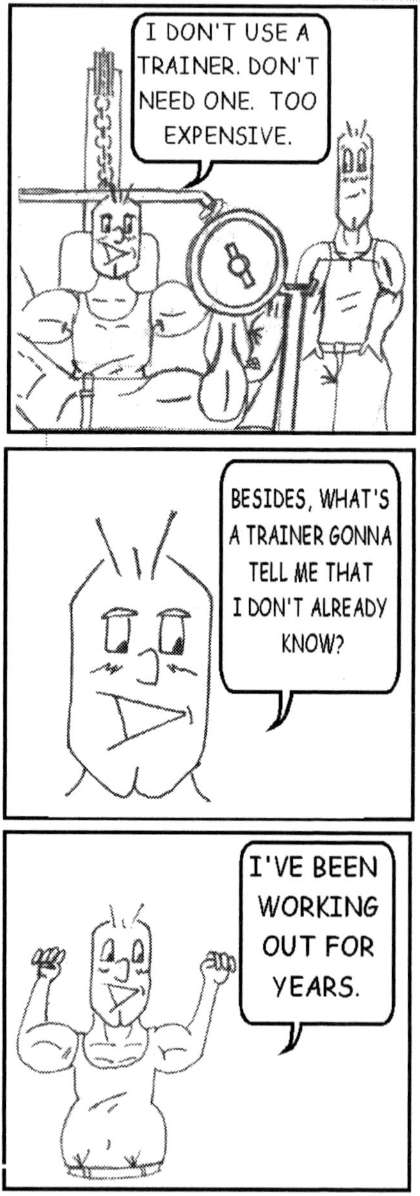

I DON'T USE A TRAINER. DON'T NEED ONE. TOO EXPENSIVE.
BESIDES, WHAT'S A TRAINER GONNA TELL ME THAT I DON'T ALREADY KNOW?
I'VE BEEN WORKING OUT FOR YEARS.

Chapter One

Sorting through the Chaos

There is considerable debate today on what it takes to be healthy and fit. Manufacturers of fitness equipment claim that their particular machine will do the job. Health clubs say that if you join their gym, the pounds will melt away. Diet books and programs claim their programs are the best for helping people lose weight and feel good about themselves. Supplement manufacturer's claim that their "pill" will help you lose weight without exercise or dieting.

Through all of these claims, it is difficult to determine what exactly the truth about being healthy is. Every product or program has a group of so-called experts to back them up with plenty of "words". These experts may range from not-so-credible celebrities to medical doctors. Who do you believe? What should you do?

You've heard the expression "words are cheap". Although words are necessary to communicate, words that really have no value are those that are based on incorrect facts or are bold-faced lies. Many experts use lots of words in the form of lengthy explanations to sway the American public..

Another way the American public is deceived is by "bits of truth". Although most agree that exercise is good for you, exercising with one particular machine is not going to do it all to make you healthy. I love it when a supplement company manufactures an outrageous claim for results and has in the fine print "effective when used in conjunction with a healthy diet and exercise program". Question: Do you need the supplement at all if you eat right and exercise? Would the results be the same?

Among all the chaos, however, there are some very credible sources trying desperately to get the message out about the right way to get fit and be healthy. These people are not trying to sell a quick fix to make a buck nor are they willing to improperly inform the public for their own gain. Their intents are true, but lost in all the misinformation.

The Purpose of this Book

We developed this book out of our own needs for a simple published piece on the basics of exercise and nutrition. The first evolution of this book covered strictly strength training for women. As we learned more about the importance of diet and exercise, we added chapters to where it is today.

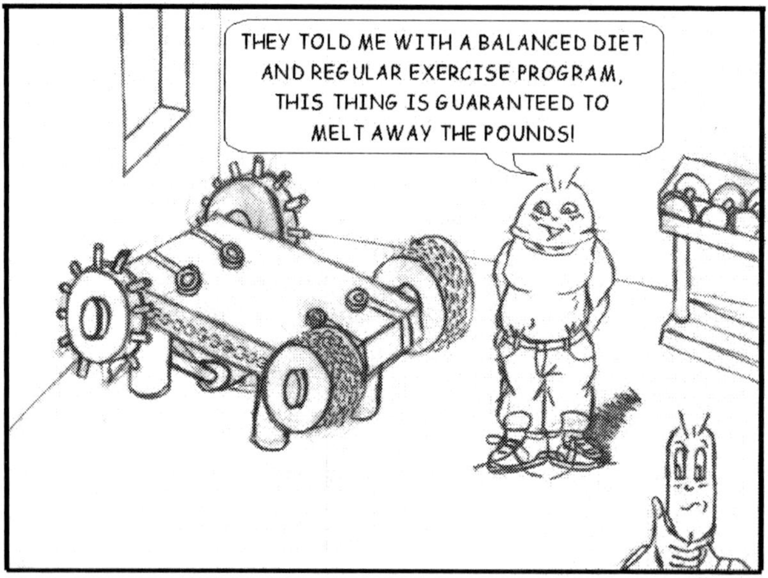
THEY TOLD ME WITH A BALANCED DIET AND REGULAR EXERCISE PROGRAM, THIS THING IS GUARANTEED TO MELT AWAY THE POUNDS!

This book was developed as an aide for our own personal trainers at Fay's Fitness. Most trainers are successful at helping you develop a safe and effective exercise program, but do not feel comfortable counseling in areas outside their area of expertise, particularly regarding nutrition. Others act more as lifestyle counselors and help you with both nutrition and exercise. This book covers the basics of an effective program and gives the trainer's client an overview of the an effective program. It in no way serves as a substitute for a trainer's knowledge.

In our experience, we have found that most of the credible sources publish similar truths when it comes to lifestyle management. This book is more of a research paper on how to get started living a healthy lifestyle rather than another "how-to" book. None of the ideas are new, and all of the concepts mentioned are based on credible sources and/or conclusive testing. This book pulls together all the basic, important information for living healthy and presents it in a format that is easy to understand.

This booklet is not about long explanations. We encourage you to read all the studies and books of some of the credible sources we have listed in the Appendix and get yourself educated on how the body works. This education goes a long way in understanding how your body works and how important it is to fuel and work your body for optimum performance. This book is to the point and will outline the means for you to design a program that will be successful based on the sources.

Another reason you should review the sources is because some of them put their own spin on what works based on the author's experience. For instance, *Body for Life* promotes interval training for the aerobic part of your plan. For those with little time to spare, this difference may make a significant change in keeping with the program. You'll be surprised at the helpful hints you'll pick up reading these sources.

Criteria for a Successful Program

There are several elements to a successful program that put you on track for a healthy lifestyle. When evaluating different programs for this booklet due consideration was paid to the following criteria. All reputable programs should be:

- Something you can live with the rest of your life. If it radically changes your lifestyle right away, it probably will not be successful long-term.
- Effective. It must work.
- Safe. No long-term problems or injuries.
- Aligned with the way nature intended.
- Self-motivating and leave you energetic. You should not feel drained, depleted, hungry or lethargic. This is not the way of a healthy human.
- Something that will add quality years to your life and "life to your years". The program must be good for your health.
- Comprehensive. All elements of your life should be considered. Balance should be the goal.

The majority of programs, plans, and equipment do not satisfy all of these criteria. Fad exercise equipment often becomes boring over time and only effects your strength <u>or</u> cardio endurance. Restrictive calorie diets leave you hungering more every day for something sweet. Diet pills, if effective, are not good to take long term. Even prescription diet pills have been pulled off the market (beware of over-the-counter pills also). So when you are looking at a program, check out how it stacks up.

The program outlined in this book meets all the guidelines. This book will focus on *physical* well being or fitness. For the *total* fitness package, however; mental and spiritual elements must be included. True happiness comes from balancing or being 'fit' in all three areas. Our discussion will be limited to the physical aspects, but due consideration must be paid to mental and spiritual elements for the total picture.

Most books and programs steer away from spiritual aspects of happiness. The only thing we will mention is that being out of balance, by not challenging yourself mentally and/or developing spiritually, will result ultimately in unhappiness. This unhappiness has been proven to effect your physical well being. Seek truth and practice it in all aspects of life.

More Tools to evaluate fitness programs

God gave us all a reasoning mind and it is within the capacity of all of us to determine what is right and what is not. As we examine data, however; we need to keep some ground rules in mind to help us with our search. These rules will help us use our minds objectively and not get thrown off course. When evaluating a new program or data:

1. **Always keep the objective in mind**. We want a healthy, long-term solution to becoming and staying fit. How will it help you meet your goals?
2. **Determine what they are they selling**. If someone offers a product or plan that seems too good to be true, determine what is for sale. In the case of products or supplements, it is simple. For diet plans, the author may be trying to sell books, but others may be selling something totally different. Some diet plans are even "selling" religion. Determining what is for sale will help you sort through the data they offer as it will give you their motive.
3. **Review the counterpoints**. For almost all plans and products, there are published counterpoints and reviews. In order to make a balanced decision, check out these reviews before you buy. Note: just because there are counterpoints, does not mean the product is poor.

Review them.

4. **Keep impulsiveness in check**. Salespeople want you to buy now because they are afraid you might make a more educated decision tomorrow.

Armed with these tools, we'll be able to navigate the swamp more successfully.

Will this Book Work for Everyone?

Sadly, the answer to this question is no.

Unfortunately, there are many individuals that will continue to look for the quick-fix. This book is not about quick-fix programs. In our opinion, there will always be a huge market for diet-pills, fad-diets, liposuction, etc. Those that are more interested in how they look or those that want to change NOW may not have the patience to do the job right. They may not be willing to change their lifestyle for total health. The other reason some will not be able to follow the guidelines in this book is because it takes work. Sorry… the body is designed to be used. If you are not getting enough activity in your life, then you will have to…here comes that terrible word…EXERCISE.

There are many who don't want to work or exercise, and though we encourage you to work into it slowly, many will not want to do even that. We ask that those who abhor exercise give it another try. Just a short walk every other day. You'll find that over time it will make you want to do it.

Chapter 2

Focus on the Big Stuff

In many fitness books, you have to search long and hard to get the gist of the information being offered. In our opinion, this contributes to our problem of being confused. In this book, we put all the essential points for developing your program in a summary at the end of each chapter. We do this for simplicity. We don't want anything to get lost in the words.

Americans fail at the big stuff when it comes to fitness - not the details. For example, the maximum intake of fat recommended in any of the credible resources is 30%. We Americans average 34%. Also, according to the Center for Disease Control (CDC), only 22% of adults engage in regular aerobic exercise. 25% of us don't exercise at all. Also, only 3 percent of all Americans meet at least four of the five federal Food Guide Pyramid recommendations for the intake of grains, fruits, vegetables, dairy products, and meats

By concentrating on the important issues, we can keep the big picture in mind. *You want a complete, well-rounded program.* I know plenty of people that spend a small fortune on expensive vitamin and mineral supplements, but do little exercise. You'll also see those that do a tremendous amount of aerobic exercise, but don't watch how they fuel their bodies. Concentrate on a creating a complete program with a focus on the major points.

The time phase list that follows will help you prioritize and change for good. There is no predetermined length of time for each phase. It could be weeks or even months depending on where you are currently. If you want faster results, make the changes quicker, but keep in mind that radical changes decrease your likelihood of sticking with the program. Old habits are hard to break.

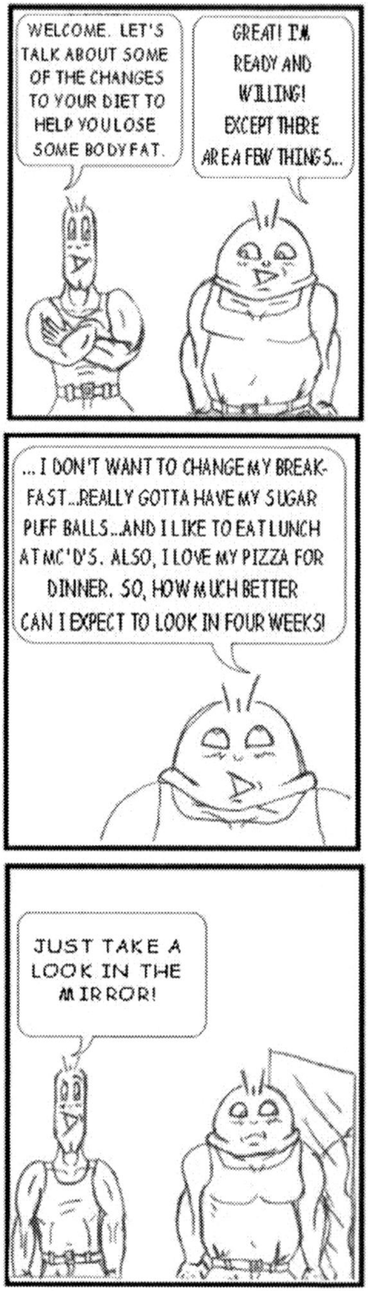
WELCOME. LET'S TALK ABOUT SOME OF THE CHANGES TO YOUR DIET TO HELP YOU LOSE SOME BODYFAT.
GREAT! I'M READY AND WILLING! EXCEPT THERE ARE A FEW THINGS...
...I DON'T WANT TO CHANGE MY BREAK-FAST...REALLY GOTTA HAVE MY SUGAR PUFF BALLS...AND I LIKE TO EAT LUNCH AT MC'D'S. ALSO, I LOVE MY PIZZA FOR DINNER. SO, HOW MUCH BETTER CAN I EXPECT TO LOOK IN FOUR WEEKS!
JUST TAKE A LOOK IN THE MIRROR!

Willingness to Change

Speaking of breaking old habits...

Your trainer will tell you that in order for you to change your body for the better, you will need to change what you do with it. Perhaps you will need to change your eating habits and/or your exercise program. These changes may include different foods, more time exercising, etc.

While designing your program, your trainer would love it if she could start with a clean slate when it comes to your daily routine. Unfortunately, this won't happen. You already have habits that control your life and a routine that you are comfortable with. Hence, instead of starting with a clean slate, a trainer must work with your existing routine to give you something you can live with and that gets results.

Changing your health will require changes in your lifestyle and habits. Doing the same thing will yield the same results, so if you want something different, you will need to change. We all know people that do the same exercises over and over and never get improved results. Chances are they could do a lot less work to just maintain.

In order to change, you have to be willing and able. Listen to your trainer and be open-minded to her suggestions. She will design a program around your habits as best she can, but you should expect to be required to change.

Time Phasing Your Program

Your trainer can help you be successful at meeting your fitness objectives. Below, we have included a typical schedule for a person whom has never exercised before. Your trainer will help design a specific program with your needs in mind.

Phase 1 –Start with a light aerobic routine.

- Goal Setting (Chapter 5): Determine where you are and where you want to be. Write down what you currently eat and how much exercise you do for a week. Write down what your specific and realistic goals are. Address aerobic capacity, strength, measurements, body fat, and flexibility. Try not to focus on weight.
- Start with 20 minutes of exercise 3 days per week. Walking is recommended. Stretch before and after.
- Compare what you eat with the guidelines above. Figure out how many calories you should eat and determine caloric content of each meal. Add a morning meal between breakfast and lunch. Make some changes (2 or 3) to get you more in line with the recommendations. Cut back on daily intake of candy, cake, donuts, etc.

(Stop cold if you can). Make sure you are getting your protein and carbohydrates.

- Log your progress.

Phase 2 – More adjustments

- Log your 30 minutes of aerobic exercise, 3 times per week.
- Go to six smaller meals a day. Tweak your diet a little more. Make 3 or 4 changes to get things a little more in line.

Phase 3 – Add more aerobic exercise

- 30 minutes, 5 times per week.
- A couple more diet adjustments. Substitute low sugar cereals made from whole grains for the Cocoa Blasts.

Phase 4 - Add Strength Training

- Once you have a regular aerobic routine, add strength training.
- Make sure your protein intake is on track. Carbohydrate sources should be whole grain and/or fresh.

Phase 5 – Final

- Track your progress and make the necessary adjustments to get in line with the program.

Exercise Myths

Women: Strength training will make me muscular or less feminine. This is one of our personal "favorites" that has kept women from working out with weights as they should. Women simply do not have the hormone testosterone to be super-muscular. The ones you see on magazine covers are either genetically predisposed, or chemically "enhanced".

Stomach exercises will help you lose fat around your stomach. Many people do lots of stomach crunches with this goal in mind, but it is simply not how it works. Stomach exercises will tone the muscles, but will not remove the fat. You'll need to either decrease calorie intake or burn more calories than you take in to affect the fat.

If I start exercising, I'll start losing weight. Maybe. Depends on many factors, like how overweight you are or how much you adjust your eating habits. With a properly balanced program, you will add muscle. This may result in a weight increase, even though you may have lost some fat.

You burn more calories if you exercise before eating. Eating after you exercise is beneficial in a few ways, however, increasing calorie expenditure is not one. You should eat after exercise to recharge glycogen levels and fuel muscle cells.

It's best to exercise in the morning. Only if that is the only time you can. No time of day has been proven to be better than another.

Exercise machines are more effective than free weights. You can get a good workout from either free weights, selectorized equipment, fit-balls, elastic bands, etc. It matters more how you use the equipment than what the equipment is for effective results.

Exercise turns fat into muscle. As we discussed in the sit-up myth, fat does not turn into muscle: fat is lost and muscle is built.

You need extra salt after perspiring heavily. After heavy exercise, you need more water and sugar than anything else. A typical meal will replenish more than one can perspire.

People with high blood pressure shouldn't lift weights. Not true. Just make sure you breath.

No pain, no gain. If a personal trainer quotes this phrase to you, find yourself another one. It is true, there may be some stiffness the next day after a good workout, however, your goal should be injury-free exercise. DO not push yourself beyond safe limits.

Chapter 3

Why aren't we healthy and what should we do about it?

The following explanations are geared toward one of the largest problems facing Americans today – being overweight. You may not have this problem – yet. We are devoting almost the entire chapter to this particular problem because it is *<u>the</u>* *major reason people decide to start a health program. If you generally find that you are not overweight or maybe you are an athlete with different issues, you should still read this chapter as it will give you perspective and knowledge for the future when things may change.*

If you're like most of us Americans, your fitness problem is that you are "overweight". Many believe that being overweight is the primary fitness issue facing this country today. *The Surgeon General's Call to Action to Prevent and Decrease Overweight and Obesity* supports this claim, as it reports that in 1999, 61% of U.S. adults were overweight. The report points out that over 300,000 deaths per year are currently associated with obesity, comparing it to over 400,000 deaths associated with cigarette smoking. Being overweight is a serious problem, but is it the problem we are trying to solve? Let's look a little closer.

Many people understand that there is a difference between being overweight and over-fat. Just because you weigh more than the height/weight chart in your doctor's office does not necessarily mean you have a health problem. Most serious body-builders with a 5% body fat composition would be overweight by these charts. On the other end of the scale, many individuals within the height/weight chart ranges may still have a dangerously high body fat percentage. Generally for inactive adults, if the height/weight chart (based on BMI) says you are overweight, you are over-fat as well. Keep in mind, however, it is the high body fat percentages that have been linked to health problems.

Being overweight or even overfat is not *the* problem, however. It is the *effect* of another bigger problem: an unhealthy lifestyle. Several lifestyle variables can effect how much fat your body stores. Nutrition, exercise, sleep, genetics, and stress are some of the major variables. How overfat you are is a function of these variables. Each one affects your body's capacity to store fat.

Fitness, by definition, is the quality or state of being mentally and physically healthy. **This is what we should be seeking: to be healthy.** It is interesting to note that Darwin's definition of being "fit" would be linked to survival. When you consider all the health related diseases that are linked to being unfit, you can see how fitness is important.

Being fit would include having strong muscles and bones, cardiovascular endurance and a balanced body composition (lean muscle vs. fat). Physical weight is typically a variable in the body composition equation, but is not by itself an indicator (more on this later). Being fit would include getting body fat composition in line where it should be, which may indeed result in a weight loss. Just keep in mind that it is not the problem—it is the result of the problem, i.e. not being healthy.

The reason we obsess about our weight is because it is a visible result of a health problem. It is a sign to the world that our physical and mental health are out of balance. As we stated, being over-fat is an effect of an unhealthy lifestyle. Some may think that if we look good with less weight, we will be fine. This is simply not how it works. The cause must be addressed instead of the symptom and changes must come from the inside-out. Changes to the exterior have little to do with the inside, and will leave you with the problem even though the effect has changed.

This is what is happening with weight loss programs today. The focus of most of the weight management programs is weight loss. Some of these programs give cursory attention to exercise. The solution to the problem, then, is to get the pounds off. And how is this performed? Through the only system that gives almost guaranteed results if followed: restrictive dieting. Cut back what you eat and you are sure to drop the pounds. If the pounds are not coming off fast enough, take in less calories by eating less or eating more foods that have no calories.

When followed, restrictive diets are successful at helping people lose weight. These diets come under question when you look at their long term track record and their impact on health. The vast majority of people on restrictive diet programs do not stick to them very long. Also, there are more radical programs, such as the high-protein diets, that put you at health risk. When the restrictive program is no longer followed, the weight usually goes back on – and then some.

Restrictive diets that cut calorie intake are a solution to the symptom of being overweight, but most of these diets cause you to lose lean muscle as well as fat. They are successful at dropping the weight, but also affect muscle mass. Keep in mind that one pound of muscle uses energy at a rate of about 20-50 calories per day for maintenance. Losing muscle reduces ability to burn calories, therefore making it harder to lose weight.

I hope you can see that "losing weight" should not be an objective. If you are over-fat, then you should replace the objective of losing weight with "losing fat". But why not encompass the total picture of fitness and set your goal to be healthy?

What's so bad about being out of shape?

So we're over-fat and inactive. What's wrong with that?

There is growing support for those that have accepted the fact that they are over-fat. The over-fat problem is so extensive in this country, that those that are over-fat are pulling together to try and change the perception of others that may look at those that are over-fat as being any less of a person.

Being prejudicial based on one's size is no different than prejudging someone based on the color of their skin, their sex, or their beliefs. For example, when someone we knew, let's call him "Ron", ballooned up to 214 pounds, it was due to many stress factors in his life. He and his wife just had a new baby, their bills were at an all-time high, and Ron had a relatively new job. The reaction to the stress was to eat and there was no time or energy for exercise. To prejudge someone for being over-fat without knowing the circumstances is just plain wrong.

On the other hand, let's not convince ourselves that being over-fat and out of shape is okay. It is not. First, it is unnatural. The root cause of being unhealthy is that we have fallen away from nature's system of keeping us fit to survive. The other reason it is not okay to be in an unhealthy condition is because of all the health risks. From the Surgeon General's Report, the following are potential health risks as a result of a unhealthy lifestyle:

- Increased risk of cardiovascular disease mortality in general and of coronary heart disease mortality.
- Increased risk of coronary heart disease.
- Increased risk of developing high blood pressure.
- Increased risk of developing non-insulin-dependent diabetes mellitus.
- Decreased ability to maintain independent living status and increased risk of falling in older adults.

These "increased risks" ignore all the other psychological benefits of being healthy, such as reducing stress and relieving symptoms of depression and anxiety.

Based on the above, no one should desire to be unhealthy and we should all strive to be as healthy as we can under the circumstances.

The roots of the problem

The body, though extremely complicated in its function, can be compared to a highly developed machine. Let's look at how developed it is:

- The human body can operate on any number of fuels. We are omnivorous mammals, which means we can eat and survive on vegetation as well as animal flesh.
- The human body is efficient and continually adjusts to its environment. If there is insufficient fuel or food, it will lower the rate at which it uses the fuel and it will store any extra fuel (as fat). If the body is not active, it will reduce capacity to perform certain functions as they are not needed. If muscle is not needed for function, it will be used up as fuel. The body is extremely efficient this way.
- The body is capable. We can run, jump, climb, lift, carry, etc. We are more versatile than any other creature on earth.

This is what we are by design: an extremely efficient, capable machine. For all the physical faults we may think we have, we are the most advanced creature to walk the earth. So why are many of us developed "machines" in the most technologically advanced country in the world becoming the "fattest" and least physically capable?

So how did we end up all being so fat?

Reason #1: We eat too much

In a natural state, animals typically eat what is available, when it is available. Prior to this century, it was pretty much the same for humans. Availability of food had a lot to do with what we ate and when we ate it. (Keep in mind there wasn't a lot of thought put into diet before this century. We didn't know near as much as we do today about a balanced diet.) The constraint on our diet was availability, not what we thought we should eat.

Availability of food is no longer a constraint to our eating habits. There is plenty to eat most everywhere in this country, not disregarding the poor. Also, we no longer have to eat what we don't like. We can eat what we want, regardless of whether we should.

Availability also affects **when** an animal eats. If an animal is hungry and there is food available, then it will eat. It will not wait for the noon hour bell. Before we became industrialized, it was pretty much the same for humans. Now, because of our jobs, meals are further apart and **bigger**. There is a constraint for us in the working world to when we eat. The boss wants us working between 8—12:00 and 1:00—5:00 PM.

The result of having an abundance of food and the time constraints on when we eat is overeating. Couple these factors with eating for "comfort" from mental and emotional stress, and you have the number one reason we are over-fat.

Reason #2: We eat the wrong things.

For us Americans, we can generally eat whatever we want, whenever we want. There are no controls on us as to when we can eat as there are in nature. We don't spend the majority of our day searching for food and how fast we can run doesn't determine how much we will eat that day.

Because we can eat what we want, when we want, our choices for food are not always balanced. The human body is very versatile in what it can use for fuel and we may choose to eat what sounds good more than what is good for us.

Conscientious dog owners know that feeding a dog table scraps is a poor practice. If you could ask a dog, they would prefer the scraps over their same old boring dog food. The problem is that table scraps, the food we eat, are not fit for a dog. Dog food is formulated to give a dog all the nutrients it needs in proper proportion. It is composed of grains, protein, etc., in the right amounts to keep your dog healthy. Feeding table scraps to a dog offsets the balance of the dog food. It also spoils a dog and the dog will end up wanting the more tastier scraps in lieu of what is good for it. The result can be a malnourished dog that may be overweight on a diet of food that is not good for it.

If you love your dog, feed them what is right for them.

Humans are no different. We need to have a diet of foods matched to our needs. We cannot always eat what tastes good to us, or we will fall into the same fate as the overweight dog with a diet of table scraps. We must control our diet because all the natural controls are absent.

In addition to having food available everywhere and eating what we want, the types of foods available are not as they were 100 years ago. Products are bleached, cooked, salted, and processed. They come complete with tons of preservatives, pesticides, etc. It is time consuming to find fresh whole-grained vegetables and breads. You may need to shop at specialty stores to find what you like and need, though larger markets are expanding their variety. Also, it takes time to read all the nutrition labels.

Reason #3: We don't have enough activity in our lives

Our level of activity has also changed dramatically in the past century. Prior to the automobile, people did a lot of walking to get around. Now, we spend a lot of time looking for the closest parking spot at the mall.

Washing machines do our clothes and our dishes. Cars transport our goods. Tractors do our farming and computer controlled machines make our products. Computer games have replaced several activities in our children's lives. All we have to do is sit back and press buttons. In fact, those that are most successful today are the ones that are the best at it. Survival of the fittest has a new twist.

So our culture has left us with all the food we want, though we may not be able to eat when we want, and literally no need for physical activity. It's easy to see why we have a problem. But there's more.

Reason #4: Many experts are misleading us.

The confusion regarding weight control is a major contributing factor to our obesity problem. The conflicting testimony of the experts is causing us to fail.

Science and mathematics are used to help us understand natural phenomenon. Scientists study natural laws and then develop theories and explanations on how things work. These theories are evaluated and then tested. If the theory is true, the model will work; if it is incorrect, the model will fail under test. This is considered in chemistry as the "acid test".

Most diet theories look good on paper, in fact we lay-people have considerable difficulty finding fault For instance, how are we going to argue with an endocrinologist on the principles of metabolism? The experts have an edge over us with this regard and they use it. They hold all the cards when it comes to explaining the "how" of things.

Many dieting theories fail the acid test with regards to safe and effective means to lose weight. For example, take the case for ephedra. Shortly after the recall of Fen-phen, ephedra came out as the new wonder drug for weight loss. The FDA is finally starting to crack down on its use, as there are serious side-effects for some users.

So what do we do?

The natural controls are no longer in place to help maintain a healthy body. Because we are in such an unnatural state with less activity and over-availability of food, we must put controls in place and discipline ourselves to these controls to be healthy. We are held captive in this culture, much like an animal is held captive in a zoo. The difference being that the zookeepers look out for the health of the animals. They control their diets and exercise them to maintain their health. Who does this for us?

We need to discover the right way to be healthy, commit to eating the right things, and get active. *The good news is once we start doing the right things our bodies will no longer desire the wrong ones.* For instance, once you take out the extra fat and sugar out of your diet and replace it with complex carbohydrates from fresh sources, your body won't crave the bad at all. Once you start to exercise, you won't want to stop! (But don't get too obsessed and addicted to it. Maintain balance.)

The Synergy of Exercise and Nutrition

1 + 1 = 3

That's a perspective about synergy. The combined effect of two elements is greater than the sum of its parts. There are examples of this all around us. Perhaps you have worked with someone on a job where the two of you were able to finish the job in less than half the time it would have taken you alone to do it.

This is how it works for nutrition and exercise. Exercise only works so well without proper nutrition and proper nutrition can only take you so far without exercise. You need both to be fit. Eating right helps you feel energized and as a result you will be able to exercise harder and longer. Proper fueling also improves your recovery as well as helps to develop muscle faster. Exercise in turn suppresses hunger and cravings for the wrong foods. It helps you sleep better and reduces your stress. Better rest helps your recovery from exercise and helps you stay motivated to eat right. It all works together.

There are many people that exercise but do not eat right. The result is that they get little or no benefit from the work they do. Their muscles can't get what they need to develop and workouts are strained. In some cases, they over-train which actually results in the body giving up muscle tissue as a source of energy. When someone approaches a fitness counselor about not getting results from an exercise program, a common solution is to "eat more and/or exercise less". Sounds backwards – but it works.

In Addition to Proper Nutrition and Exercise:

We have focused on the two main ingredients for a healthy lifestyle—nutrition and exercise. Generally, these are the two that are most frequently addressed, but there are others that deserve attention.

Rest. Adequate sleep and rest are critical for good health. Even if you are eating right and exercise, if you do not get proper rest, your health will suffer serious consequences. The benefits of proper nutrition and exercise will be diminished by inadequate rest. Proper nutrition and exercise will help you get the proper rest you need, but you must give yourself time to "recharge your battery". This recharging consists of Human Growth Hormone being released during our deepest level of sleep. This hormone is essential for recovery and stimulates the breakdown of fat. It also improves our immune cell function.

Stress. Mental stress greatly affects your well-being. There are many health related diseases that are caused by stress. Proper nutrition and exercise will help reduce stress, but you must also make a conscious effort to remove stress from your life. Seek out stress management skills and apply them.

Over-training

Your body has a total concept of energy that involves a cycle. Your **energy cycle** consists of three parts: activity, fatigue and recovery.

Activity. During strenuous activity, muscles rely on complex carbohydrates and oxygen. Similar to how gas is used for automobiles, complex carbohydrates offer the body energy to accomplish certain activities. Lactic acid is a by-product of carbohydrate metabolism. Lactic acid can cause fatigue and muscle soreness if not removed by oxygen.

Fatigue. When the cardiovascular system cannot meet the demands of supplying oxygen, the body becomes fatigued. Lack of energy can result when the intensity and length of activity exceeds the body's resources. When you start a new activity, you may become easily fatigued until your body adapts to a new level of energy. When you become fatigued, do not push yourself!

Recovery. Recovery doesn't necessarily occur only when you stop the activity. It takes your body 24-48 hours to recover from a strenuous workout. Working out too hard and too soon can harm your progress. The key here is not to push too hard. Enjoy your workout.

If intensity is too high, and/or there is insufficient rest between workouts, you may exhibit signs of over-training. This will not typically be a problem for those who workout three times a week for an hour or so.

Energy is a cycle of activity, fatigue and recovery. When we fail to allow adequate time for recovery, we may begin to notice a decline in our level of performance—not only in sports but in everyday activities. Knowing the symptoms of overtraining can help you recognize when it's time to take a break and give your body time to recuperate. If you recognize any of the following warning signs, take a few days off from your normal activity to evaluate your training schedule and give yourself a chance to recover your energy.

Warning Signs of Overtraining:

- Elevated resting heart rate
- Persistent Muscle Soreness
- Chronic Fatigue
- Decline in performance
- Excessive thirst
- Unexplained weight loss
- Irritability
- Loss of appetite
- More colds and infections
- Changes in sleep patterns
- Lack of menstruation

If symptoms persist

Each of the symptoms listed may be associated with other physical conditions unrelated to overtraining. If your symptoms persist after three days of recovery, call your physician, who can rule out other medical reasons for your problem.

Summary – Chapter Three

- All of us should target being healthy as our primary fitness goal.
- The majority of us Americans are unhealthy because we are less active than ever, eat too much of the wrong foods, and are misled by the experts.
- Being out of shape is not good. The acceptance of being unfit means you are willing to accept the consequences of poor health.
- Look for ways to reduce stress and get proper rest.

- Don't push too hard. Recognize the symptoms of over-training.

Activity, Fatigue and Recovery

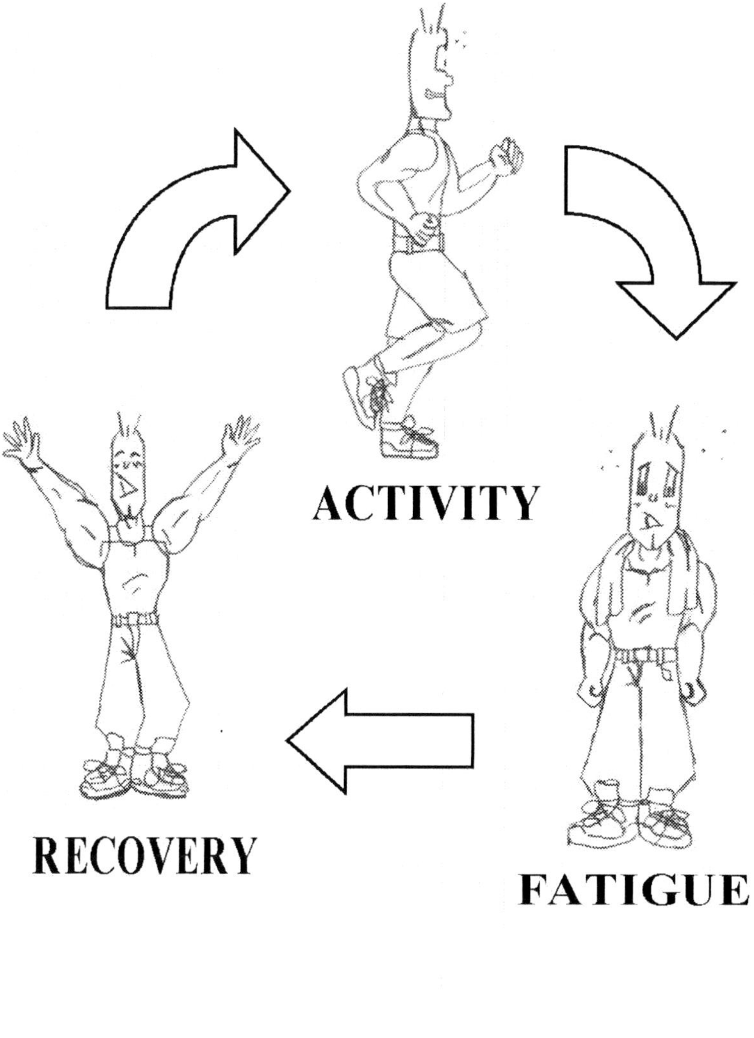

Chapter 4

Measuring Health

Before we map out our plan to get fit, we need to know where we are and where we are heading. In this chapter, we will spend some time thinking about what being healthy actually is. Once we have established this goal, developing our plan will be possible.

We all agree that a healthy body will:

- Be physically capable. The body should be able to perform physical tasks, such as run, walk, lift, pull, push, etc., at a level it was designed for, naturally.
- Not be prone to disease and illness. It should have a strong immune system and should live a long time.
- Be comprised of strong bones, tendons, ligaments as well as strong muscles. It should not be prone to injury under physical stress.
- Have energy. It will not be lethargic and drained. It will feel rested and prepared.
- Have endurance. It will be able to bear extended periods of aerobic exhilaration.

It's interesting to note that many of the diet programs today ignore the goal of having a healthy body in lieu of losing weight. Restrictive diets can make you prone to illness, make you feel tired, and do little to develop your strength and endurance.

With the goal of being healthy, we will need to take inventory of some of the gages available to measure how healthy we are. These gages will establish a baseline and mark our prog??ress as we go. Because everyone is different, the "readings" on our gages will be unique for each person. Factors such as age, frame size, sex, genetics, etc., all come in to play. If we were all the same, we could say that everyone should be able to run a 6-minute mile. Because of our differences, this is not practical.

With so many different ways to measure health, your personal trainer becomes an invaluable asset in selection and application of the tools available. She can help you determine exactly where you stand. Here are some things she will look:

How You Feel

The best gage in determining if you are healthy is *how you feel*. If you are healthy, you will feel energized and alive. You will be motivated and positive. This feeling will last throughout your waking hours (not just show up when you wake-up and then disappear a couple of hours into your workday). You should have spring in your step and be ready to take on the world.

Bring it on!

If you don't feel this way, well, that's what we're here for...

Body Composition

The CDC and the Surgeon General correlate physical fitness with how much body fat you have. Chances are, if your body fat is too high, you're out of shape and susceptible to many of the illnesses associated with being overfat.

Body composition is much more accurate for determining whether you are "too heavy" than the traditional height vs. weight charts. As mentioned, many athletes and bodybuilders would be considered overweight by the old charts. This is because most height vs. weight charts do not consider *body composition*, or how much of the body is fat and how much is lean muscle. People with large developed muscles, like athletes, will weigh more. Does this mean they should be concerned about being overweight?

Not at all. Just because the chart indicates someone is overweight, does not necessarily mean they are unhealthy. The real concern is with the *amount or percentage of the body that is fat.*

As we learned, excessive body fat is a health risk. High body fat composition has been linked to an increased risk of heart disease, diabetes, stroke, cancer and other diseases. So how fat is overfat?

Percent Body Fat Composition - Recommended Ranges

(Based on St. Jude's Health Connection Seminar, 1997 and findings from Lohman, Houtkooper and Going in ACSM's *Health and Fitness Journal*, Jan.-Feb., 1997)

There are several ways to measure body fat. Your trainer will be able to help you with this and will employ one of several methods. Some use either skin-fold calipers or a device that uses bioelectrical impedance. Either of these methods provides a good means to establish a baseline for monitoring results. It is not a good practice, however, to use the methods interchangeably. Sticking with one method, and preferably one person is the best practice.

The most accurate body fat analysis is by hydrostatic testing. This is not typically practical, as it is expensive, not readily available, and time consuming. DEXA scanning is also accurate. This test - designed for osteoporosis – can give accurate body fat percentage as well.

Another simple means of determining potential health risks associated with body fat is with waist and hip measurements. Calculate your waist-to-hip ratio by dividing your waist measurement by your hip measurement. Health risks for women increase with a waist-to-hip ratio of over .86. For men, health risks are associated with waist-to-hip ratios over .95.

% Body Fat Ranges for Good Health

FEMALE

Age Group	19-24	25-29	30-34	35-39	40-44	45-49	50-59	60+
Min %	12	12	16	16	16	20	20	20
Max %	21.9	22.4	22.7	23.7	25.4	27.2	30	30.8

MALE

Age Group	19-24	25-29	30-34	35-39	40-44	45-49	50-59	60+
Min %	5	5	7	7	7	7	9	9
Max %	14.8	16.5	18	19.4	20.5	21.5	22.7	23.5

As discussed, how much someone weighs is a poor indicator of health. If you are trying to determine if you are losing fat, use one of the means discussed; have your trainer do an analysis or take your measurements. Another simple way to find out if you are losing fat is is how your clothes fit. If your clothes are getting looser, chances are you are losing fat. Don't focus on the scale.

Aerobic Capacity

Cardiovascular health refers to the condition of the respiratory and circulatory systems of the body, namely the heart, lungs and blood vessels. Good cardio health is associated with having good endurance during aerobic activities. Developing cardiovascular health requires aerobic exercise. Aerobic exercises such as walking, cycling and swimming stress the heart muscle, thereby making it stronger and increasing its efficiency as a pump. Aerobic means oxygen is used - you breathe harder doing the exercises, as the body requires more oxygen to supply the energy.

Your Resting Heart Rate (RHR) is an indicator of cardiovascular health. As the heart's efficiency to pump increases, your resting heart rate should go down. Your resting heart rate is counted in the AM before getting out of bed. A normal heart rate is between 60 and 100 beats per minute (bpm). Generally, the lower the better (healthier). Trained athletes will have a resting heart rate of 40-60 bpm.

Blood pressure is another indicator of cardiovascular health. Normal blood pressure is considered 120/80. If you are over 140/90 consistently, a doctor should monitor it. As your heart becomes more efficient, blood pressure will go down.

If you smoke, becoming a non-smoker is the single best thing you can do for your cardio health. Smoking makes the heart work harder, increases heart rate and blood pressure, as well as making you more prone to illness. This is not to mention the effects of second hand smoke on those around you. It's interesting to note that living a sedentary lifestyle gives you the same health risk as smoking one pack per day of cigarettes.

Aerobic capacity can be measured by using a **three-minute submaximum step** test protocol. This test was developed for the YMCA and assesses Recovery Heart Rate. The quicker your heart rate comes down after exercising vigorously, the better shape you are in. Your trainer may perform this test typically to determine where you are regarding cardiovascular health. The test allows the trainer to design an aerobic program of appropriate intensity.

A simple indicator of cardio health is how you feel after vigorous exercise. If you can walk for 45 minutes at a brisk pace without getting tired, chances are you are in pretty good shape. On the other hand, if you do not feel energized after a walk, you will need more focus on your cardio training.

Strength

Strength is the ability of the muscles to lift or oppose resistance. Even though we are all not Olympic athletes, being strong is important to everyone. Strength training, also referred to as weight or resistance training, is required to increase muscular strength. It differs from aerobic exercise, in that the focus is not to primarily develop cardio-respiratory endurance (CRE). To effectively develop CRE requires consistent vigorous activity for 20 minutes or more. Strength training requires short bursts of energy, which are not usually maintained for any prolonged period. Strength training is a form of anaerobic exercise (without oxygen) as energy is supplied through stored carbohydrates.

Flexibility

Flexibility refers to the range of motion of the body's joints and muscles. Stretching exercises increase flexibility, thereby decreasing risk of injury to the joints, bones, ligaments, and tendons, as well as increasing the range of motion. Stretching also increases blood flow to the muscles.

Your trainer may do a sit and reach test to measure flexibility in your hamstrings and lower back muscles. This is a simple stretch test that can be representative of overall flexibility.

Other Measures

The gages above bring science and measurement to getting fit. There are plenty of other ways to measure your progress.

- How long you can keep up a given aerobic activity. Many people getting back into shape use this method for marking progress. Maybe they start with 10 minutes of activity and work their way up to 30 minutes.
- Timing distance covered during a walk, jog or bike. If you can make a specified distance in less time, you are

getting better conditioned.

When using these methods, always stay within your target heart rate zone.

Summary – Chapter Four

- How you feel is the best gage for measuring your health.
- Body composition is the best way to determine if you are overweight. Body fat measurements over 35% are unhealthy
- Aerobic exercise promotes cardiovascular health. Three-minute step test, resting heart rate, and blood pressure (Normal = 120/80) are measures of cardio health.
- Strength and flexibility are measurable, but are very individualistic.
- If you smoke, becoming a non-smoker is the single best thing you can do for your health.
- If you are overweight, focus on fat-loss rather than weight loss.

Chapter 5

Setting Goals

Goal setting is very important because 1) it gives you a target to shoot for and 2) achieving your goals will help motivate you to do more. Once you've started an exercise routine, goal setting is an effective way to keep you pumped up. Having specific long-term and short-term goals will serve as motivation to get you where you want to be.

Many people start out with general goals like 'to get in shape' or 'lose a few pounds'. Two very important points about proper goal setting are 1) be specific and 2) write them down.

Helping people set reasonable goals and then mapping out a plan to achieve them is one of the big reasons for hiring a personal trainer. Tracking progress is sometimes difficult, but a trainer realizes the importance and will spend the time to ensure progress is recorded and their clients are on track.

From Zig Zigler's *See You at the Top*, an effective method of setting goals is as follows:

- *Step One* – Identify your goals. What do you wish to accomplish?
- *Step Two* – Identify the benefits of reaching this goal. This will determine your motivation.
- *Step Three* – Identify major obstacles to overcome. What will keep you from reaching your goal? Also, identify what pain you will have if you do not reach your goal.
- *Step Four* – Determine the skills or knowledge you need to meet the goal.

- *Step Five* – Identify resources you have available to reach your goal. Who or what can help?
- *Step Six* – Develop a plan of action to reach the goal.
- *Step Seven* – Set a date for completion.

Step One - Identify your goals.

Here are some goals to address:

- To be healthy and feel good. Focus should not be on how you look or how much you weigh at the expense of your health. If you are over-fat, focus on body composition.
- Develop a plan you can stick with. You want to develop a plan you can stick to for a lifetime.
- Cardiovascular goal. Everyone's will be different. Some may just want to be able to walk up a flight of stairs without getting winded. Others may set out to do their first half-marathon.
- Strength goals. Set goals for what weights and repetitions you should be working with.
- Nutrition: What do you need to improve? What do you need to eat more or less of?

Some people start exercising with a short-term goal in mind like shaping up after having a baby. This is fine, but as we discussed, exercise should be a lifetime commitment. The goal set when you started should be expanded into a long-term goal of keeping fit.

The best motivation for training is realizing results. As you start feeling better and see improvement, you will be driven to continue. For example, if you consistently strength train 2-3 times a week, you should see and feel visible changes after one month. Perhaps not a loss of weight, but a shift in muscle/fat ratio. Your muscles will be stronger, firmer and shapelier. You may notice your clothes fitting better and the loss of inches. You may also realize what a great stress reducer weight training is and how you have gained a more positive outlook.

Set specific long-range goals. Write down what you expect from your program. If you're exercising for fat loss, how much do you want to lose? How strong do you want to be? How many miles do you want to be able to walk without tiring and in what length of time? Be realistic and write down where you are now and where you expect to be.

Set specific short-term goals. Now that you know where you want to be, break up the big goal into smaller parts. For instance, if you want to lose 20 pounds in 6 months, try losing 3-4 pounds per month. (Realistic goal for fat loss is 1-2 pounds per week.) As you lose, you will become more motivated to achieve.

Once again, it is important to write these things down! If it is not written down, three months from when you started you will question your progress. The only way motivation can be derived from this process is by knowing where you have been and where you want to be. Keep a planner or log to document your routine and progress.

As you continue to train, the results may not be so evident. Just because it is not visually apparent in a mirror does not mean you are not getting results. This is why it is necessary to keep an accurate record of your condition. You should record the weight you workout with along with the number of reps and sets. Also, keep track of all your measurements and weight, at least on a monthly basis. This way even if your results are not visible to the eye, you will still 'see' improvement. Write down how you feel mentally: increased energy, more positive, sleeping better, etc. Use your training journal to record your results. Keep a food diary or other fitness related records in a notebook as well. It is not important how you do it only that you do.

Step Two - Benefits of reaching this goal

Experience has shown that those with a regular exercise routine, such as walking or aerobics, are much more successful in starting and keeping with a strength training program. But what if you don't have a routine? How do you muster up enough energy to get started?

You need to ask yourself: Why do I want to be fit and how bad do I want it?

You know there are a host of good reasons for everyone to exercise, namely to:

- Improve quality of life..
- Improve appearance.
- Lengthen our lives.
- Enable us to do more.
- Reduce stress

You'd think these reasons by themselves would be enough, but they are not typically the reasons someone starts a health program. Some people start so they will look good to go on a cruise or for summer or to prepare for a class reunion. Even though the aforementioned reasons should prevail, you need to dig deep to find out why you personally want or need an exercise routine in your life.

People with busy schedules may think they simply do not have the 20-30 minutes, three times a week to exercise. Exercise does not have a high priority in their lives, and is neglected. After a few years of not being in shape, the thought of the 'long road ahead' to get fit is enough to deter one from even starting an exercise routine. Consider the following:

All the benefits of being fit have been covered and you know it is important. Treat it that way when you schedule your life. People work out anywhere from 5:00 AM to 10:00 PM to get it into their schedule. When you understand the importance of exercise, no schedule is too tight to work in 20 to 30 minutes three times a week. (The Surgeon General now advises 30 minutes of exercise most days of the week.)

Don't start something you can't commit to long-term. Exercise must be enjoyable and more importantly consistent. It must become routine. What kind of exercise would you enjoy doing all the time? For many people the answer is walking. People walk in the early hours, at lunch and after dinner to get exercise. Would one of these times work for you?

You'll also want to use this step to consider what will be painful about not working toward and achieving your goal. Examples: low energy, health problems, needing larger sized clothes, etc.

You must recognize the importance of exercise and give it a priority. Once the priority is established, the next step should be to start with a simple aerobic routine that you enjoy doing to develop a habit. Crawl before you walk; walk before you run..

Step Three - Identify major obstacles to overcome

What stands in your way of getting healthy? In our experience, the big reasons are:

- Family and work obligations. Fitness becomes a low priority next to these.
- Education and knowledge. In many cases it is just a matter of knowing the right way to get fit.
- Procrastination and lack of motivation. People that are not active and don't eat right are typically less energetic and motivated than those that do. In physics, it is referred to as "static friction". It takes more energy to

get something started than to keep it moving.

- Lack of equipment.
- Despise exercising.
- A closed mind. People that are not open to change, may not.
- Weather. It can really put a crunch on an outdoor walking or biking program.

Think carefully about the reasons you have started and stopped a program in the past.

Step Four - Identify skills or knowledge you need to meet the goal.

This book will help you get on the right track, but it contains only a portion of what you need. You will need more guidance regarding specifics of your individual diet and exercise program. ***This is where your trainer can help.*** Also, we encourage you to read some of the resources referenced in the back to expand your knowledge.

Step Five - Identify other resources you have available to reach your goal.

Look back at the obstacles to overcome. What will help you deal with these? Some suggestions:

- Work with a personal trainer. They have high success rates and are well worth the money, when you consider what they do for you.
- Work with your doctor, a dietitian and/or a physical therapist if you have specific concerns.
- Open your mind to change. Try something new and different. Perhaps an activity you haven't done in a while or maybe something totally new.
- Exercise with a buddy. They will encourage you and make it fun. A partner will push you on the days you do

not feel like exercising, as you will push them when they do not feel up to it. Having someone to workout with also makes it more fun and if you enjoy what you are doing you are more apt to stick with it.

- Join a support group.
- Read some of the books in the Appendix. Get educated on what it takes to get fit.
- Get some equipment to exercise with or join a gym. An indoor bike or treadmill will help on those rainy and snowy days. Fitballs and exercise tubing are another way to incorporate stability and resistance training at home.

Step Six – Develop your plan.

In the next chapters, we will provide you with the elements to be included in your plan. As you know by now, we will address nutrition, aerobic exercise and strength training.

The first part of your plan will be to review what you eat and how much. Compare what you learn in this chapter to your current habits. Make adjustments accordingly.

The next step will be development of your cardiovascular training. Typically, the core of your exercise program should start with aerobic exercise; however, there are exceptions to this rule. Those that are not mobile due to age or obesity may want to start off with strength training and build up to a point where they can do some aerobic exercise. Your program should start with walking, biking, cross-country skiing swimming, or whatever suits you. Remember to stretch as a part of your warm up and also as part of your cool down. This will help meet your flexibility needs.

Once you get started, there are several ways to maintain and increase your motivation and drive to exercise.

Step Seven – Identify a completion date for your short-

term goal.

To develop a habit, it takes at least three months. Set a realistic goal with your trainer for 12-13 weeks from now, addressing the adjustments you want to make in your lifestyle to get healthy. Address nutrition and exercise specifically.

The key will be to make the goals realistic and attainable. This will help with your motivation.

Backsliding

Very few people have started an exercise and nutrition program and have not slipped back into old habits now and then. Most of us experience some backsliding along the way. The key is to learn from each backsliding incident to help prevent it in the future.

Find the reason for the lapse. Some common causes are:

- Force of habit
- Stress
- Boredom
- Discouragement with slow progress
- Social situations
- Impulse eating
- Lack of self-confidence

When you discover the reason for the lapse, think of ways to avoid it in the future.

Diet counselors recommend rehearsing appropriate responses to the situations that tempt us to backslide. Such responses could include any of the following:

- Wait 10 minutes before eating;
- Recite a list (written in advance) of the advantages of not giving in;
- Reward yourself in a specific way for not giving in;
- Call a friend for support.

Never underestimate the force of habit. Identify the destructive habits and then try to work out of them or work them into healthy alternatives. If you normally have a Snickers bar in the afternoon, try a healthier meal replacement bar..

What are the different reasons you backslide? List your vulnerable points and practice a response to them. For instance, if boredom causes you to backslide, make a list of activities to overcome boredom: take a walk, write a letter, or treat yourself to a facial, get new music or an exercise video. Give yourself some positive feedback for your successes. Keep the phone number of a supportive friend handy for when you feel weak.

If conflict with a family member or spouse triggers backsliding, get outside help. Above all, don't give up. Everyone backslides sometimes. Treat backsliding episodes as opportunities to learn from your mistakes. Talk to a counselor, pastor or healthcare provider about working out problems that may lead to backsliding in your diet.

Fitting Activity In Your Busy Schedule

You know that becoming physically fit can enhance the quality—and number—of the years ahead. Perhaps you can't seem to find enough time to make fitness work for you. Making time for fitness means setting priorities, sneaking extra activities into daily routines and scheduling fitness time as you would other important events.

Fitness needs to be a priority. Ask an expectant parent about the preferred gender of their baby-to-be. The typical answer? "It doesn't matter, as long as the baby is healthy." Health is the most precious quality we can wish for a newcomer into the world, and deciding to stay fit and healthy is our way of protecting that gift. You can become more fit by exercising just 20 to 30 minutes, three times a week. Isn't it worth your time to make fitness a priority in your life?

Schedule your fitness time as you would an important meeting. Many business people have traded the "business lunch" for an exercise session at the gym. Why not mix business with pleasure? Take a brisk walk during your lunch hour or, instead of a coffee break, try a stretch break. Rather than joining friends for drinks after work, get together for a game of softball, racquetball or a vigorous hike. Whatever you do, stick to that scheduled activity.

There's every reason to do something good for yourself by making fitness one of your daily priorities. By setting aside just 20 to 30 minutes, three times a week for vigorous activity, and by sneaking extra activity into your daily routines, you can become fitter, happier and more productive.

As you consider your goals...

Discover what your motivation is. Think about your reason for wanting to get in shape. Is it enough to support a long range commitment. Are you dieting to get ready for the swimsuit season or because your doctor told you your next heart attack could be fatal? Weight loss that is permanent is more often the result of long-term health considerations than of short-term goals such as the upcoming class reunion.

Are your goals realistic? Perhaps the major reason diets fail is the dieter hopes to shed a large amount of weight in a hurry and get quick results. As discussed, quick-fix programs which are difficult to stick with may result in achieving the short-term goal of losing weight; however, the person on the program will eventually resume her old habits. If you expect to lose more than one or two pounds a week, you're setting yourself up for failure. Expecting a diet to be a temporary measure rather than a life-long change in eating and exercise habits is also a surefire way to fail.

Will you have support of others? Surround yourself with a network of supportive people. Tell these people what you need from them to help you. Have them cheer you on, nag you when you lapse, or just leave you alone. Prevent them from bringing food into the house that will sabotage your self-will. Talk over your plans with your family. Let them know how important it is to you. You'll need their support.

Summary

- If you have had difficulty in the past sticking with a good program consider consulting a personal trainer. They will help with your training, and help you deal with the psychological issues that may keep you from being successful.
- Goal setting is an effective method to assist with getting in shape. **Goals should be written down and progress should be tracked.** This will motivate you.
- Backsliding is natural. Use it to learn ways to cope in the future.
- Make fitness a priority!
- One of your goals should be to form a lifetime habit of eating right and exercise.

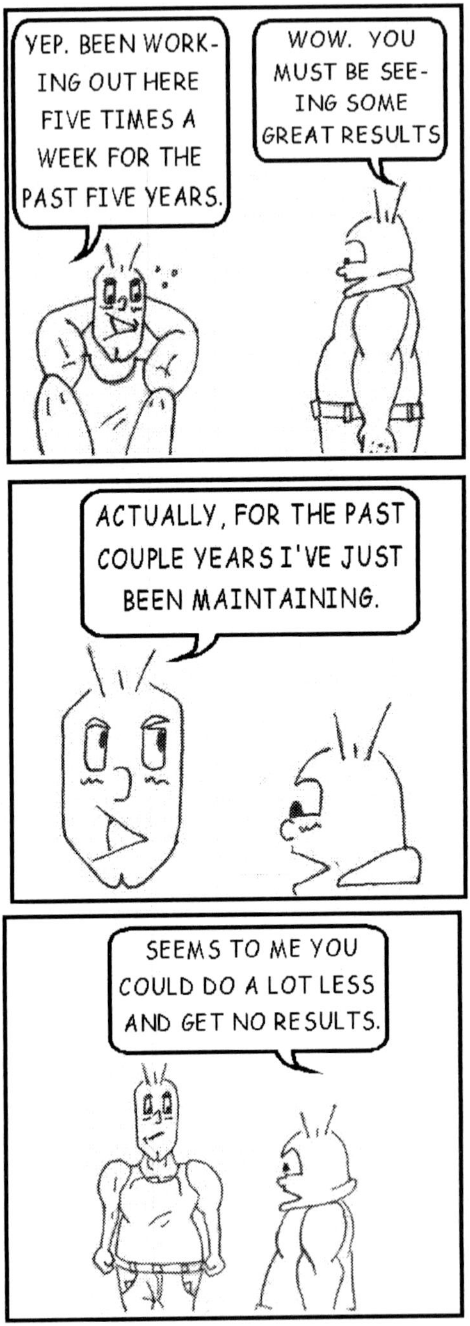
YEP. BEEN WORK-ING OUT HERE FIVE TIMES A WEEK FOR THE PAST FIVE YEARS.
WOW. YOU MUST BE SEE-ING SOME GREAT RESULTS
ACTUALLY, FOR THE PAST COUPLE YEARS I'VE JUST BEEN MAINTAINING.
SEEMS TO ME YOU COULD DO A LOT LESS AND GET NO RESULTS.

Chapter 6

Eating Right

Nutrition is a science. To totally understand what we should eat would require years of study. But what do we need to know to get our nutrition on track to be healthy? Do we need all the specifics of how food is converted to energy? Absolutely not.

At this point, we understand that exercise and proper nutrition work together for good health. You will only get a fraction of the benefit of your exercise program without proper nutrition and proper nutrition will not realize its full effect on you without exercise.

Want details? There are plenty of good references. We recommend *Strong Women Eat Well* by Miriam Nelson. It is an excellent resource. We also recommend *Transform!* by Phil Kaplan.

As we mentioned, many people tend to miss the big things while focusing on the details. Listed are the major concerns with your nutrition plan.

Balancing Carbs, Protein, and Fat

There are six nutrients that are essential for life: protein, carbohydrates, fats, water, vitamins, and minerals. The nutrients with calories; such as carbohydrates, proteins and fats, should be balanced. Here's the recommended ranges according to the Recommended Dietary Allowance (RDA):

Carbohydrates: 55-60%
Protein: 12-20%
Fat: < 30%. Below 10% of saturated fats

There can be some adjustment to these ranges. Kaplan recommends the following to keep energy levels high, adequately fuel metabolism, and keep body fat levels controlled:

Carbohydrates: 60-65%
Protein: 20-25%
Fat: < 15%, limited to 5% saturated

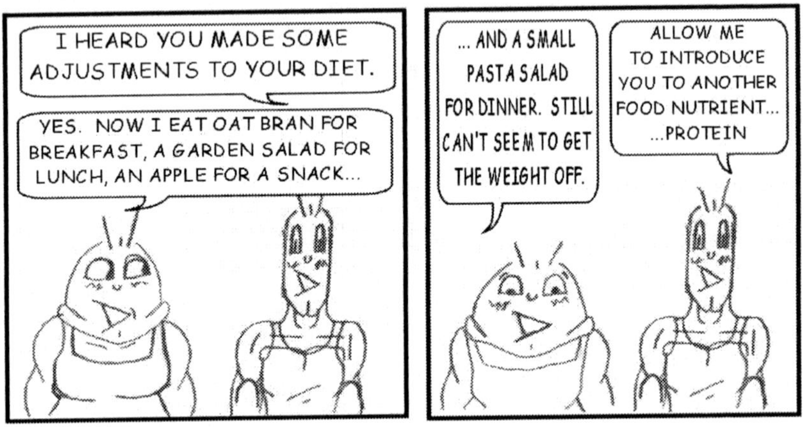
I HEARD YOU MADE SOME ADJUSTMENTS TO YOUR DIET.
YES. NOW I EAT OAT BRAN FOR BREAKFAST, A GARDEN SALAD FOR LUNCH, AN APPLE FOR A SNACK...
... AND A SMALL PASTA SALAD FOR DINNER. STILL CAN'T SEEM TO GET THE WEIGHT OFF.
ALLOW ME TO INTRODUCE YOU TO ANOTHER FOOD NUTRIENT... ...PROTEIN

Try to balance each of your meals within the ranges listed. Keep in mind, however, that there are 9 calories per gram of fat and 4 calories per gram of carbohydrate and protein. One way to make your figuring easy, try dividing your plate ½ vegetables, ¼ protein and ¼ grains/complex carbohydrates. Plates are available that have dividers with these proportions built-in.

Since all of these nutrients are essential, diets that restrict food groups and/or drastically reduce calories are generally not healthy long term. They throw off our body balance. When previous eating patterns are resumed, weight is usually gained back. At this point, muscle has been lost and fat is gained, creating a less desirable body composition.

Make a log of what you eat every day and see how your percentages stack up. <u>Read the nutrition facts labels of what you eat.</u> We have included a chart in the Appendix of some foods that typically do not have nutritional labels, such as fresh fruits and meats. You can also check out **www.nutri-facts.com**. Once you have made the adjustments to your meals to get the correct proportions, then you don't have to keep track of it as diligently.

Protein: Protein is used to maintain and build any type of cellular tissue. If you are overweight, you might want to shift your fats to the lower limit and your protein to the upper, but don't exceed 30% protein. Lean protein sources should come from egg whites, chicken, turkey, fish and seafood. Limit red meat to lean cuts and use sparingly due to saturated fat content. Lean dairy options include skim milk, non-fat/low-fat yogurt and cottage cheese. Strive for 2-3 servings per day for calcium intake.

Vegetable protein includes soy, lentils, beans, and nuts. However, vegetable proteins do not supply complete essential amino acids in a single source, so must be combined with other complementary protein vegetable sources. Examples include lentils with whole grains or brown rice with black beans. Avoid processed, refined products as amino acids can be depleted in process. If you are using incomplete protein sources such as these, you will have to carefully monitor which amino acids they have to ensure you get the complete sets. Most vegetarians are well educated on the concept of "complementary" proteins, however, it can be difficult.

Nuts are high in fat (though it is "good fat") so limit intake. Use nuts to replace foods in your diet, rather than adding them. Soy is a complete protein, however, safe limits have not been established. It is still under study in regards to perimenopausal and menopausal women. It has been shown to increase thyroid hormonal levels. A handful of soy nuts per day has been shown to be beneficial.

There is no scientific evidence that having over 15% of your calories come from protein has any benefit for muscle building. There may be other benefits, however, to increasing protein intake to above 15% if you are trying to lose weight. Many of these benefits have not been proven, but are supported with some of our credible sources. 30% is the upper limit on protein intake, as more than this has been linked to serious health problems.

Spread your protein intake throughout the day. Strive to have some with each meal.

Carbohydrate Sources: Carbohydrates are used for energy. *There are both complex and simple sources.* Complex carbs include fresh, whole grained sources and fresh fruit and vegetables. Examples of grain sources: 100% whole wheat in breads, crackers and pasta, brown rice, potatoes, oatmeal, couscous, bulgar, millet, and buckwheat. Fresh fruits and vegetables are better than processed (canned). Whole grain is better than refined white flour (even if enriched). Complex carbs provide us with fiber (soluble and insoluble) to keep our digestive system health, and prevent disease.

It takes the body longer to break down complex carbohydrates into glucose, so blood sugar levels rise slowly after eating these. Carbohydrates are also broken down and stored as glycogen in the muscles. This provides the energy for your workouts. If it is not used up, it is converted to fat.

Intake of refined sugar, though a carbohydrate, should be moderated, particularly if you are overweight. Sugar is a simple carbohydrate. Sucrose is the common table sugar and is broken down very quickly to glucose. This causes a quick rise in blood sugar levels, which is followed by a quick rise in insulin to act on this. The "sugar rush" quickly becomes the "sugar crash". You then crave more sugar and the cycle continues. This roller coaster ride leads to increased sugar cravings, increased body fat, and insulin resistance that could ultimately result in development of Type II diabetes. It is best to avoid refined sugar in many of its forms (cookies, cakes, candies, etc.). Read labels – sugar sources often end in –"ose" maltose, dextrose, etc.

Though sugar is not good as a snack or meal, it does have a place. It is beneficial after heavy aerobic exercise to restore glycogen levels. Check out the major ingredients of sports drinks – mostly sugar-water. Follow these sugar snacks with a complex carbohydrate and protein to moderate your blood sugar. Also, honey and molasses are healthier alternative sources to refined sugar.

Fat is an essential part of our brain and nervous system. Fat acts as an insulator; protector of our organs and is an energy reserve. Dietary fat is essential but needs to be limited to the proportions previously discussed. Dietary fat increases cholesterol, which can lead to heart disease. Desirable total cholesterol is below 200 mg/dl.

There are three types of fat: saturated, monounsaturated, and polyunsaturated. Saturated fat is solid at room temperature and so is harder to break down. Sources include animal fat, coconut and palm oils, butter, and mayonnaise. Hydrogenated or partially hydrogenated oil, a source of trans fat, acts the same as saturated fats. These need to be limited. Saturated fat increases LDL (Bad cholesterol). Normal level is below 130 mg/dl. You'll find trans fat appearing on more and more nutrition labels.

Monounsaturated fat includes canola oil, peanut oil, and virgin olive oil. These are preferable as they lower LDL without affecting HDL (good cholesterol). Normal HDL is above 60 mg/dl. Below 35 mg/dl is not healthy.

Polyunsaturated fats include safflower, sunflower and corn oils. These lower LDL, but also lower HDL. Fish oils, a polyunsaturated oil and Omega 3 fatty acid, are found in fatty fish like tuna and salmon. It's also available as a supplement and has been found to prevent heart disease. *To lower your LDL, cut your saturated fat intake. To increase your HDL, increase your aerobic exercise.*

Supplementation

Supplementation of vitamins and minerals may be essential, depending on your diet. Vitamins assist in metabolic processes. Minerals combine to form enzymes, hormones, and body structures. They do not provide energy. A multivitamin/mineral doesn't hurt; however, if you are eating 5-9 daily servings of fresh fruits and vegetables, you may not need it. Vitamins C and E and calcium are typically advised, though E has been coming under fire lately.

Meal supplements. Though not necessary, meal replacements may help balance out meals. These are replacements – not additions. Look for products within the calorie percentages above. Avoid high protein bars and weight gain products, which have incorrect balance. If you are low on protein for a particular meal, then a protein shake may work for you, especially if you are unable to cook a meal on the run.

Some very important points:

Drink lots of water. 8-10 cups of water per day is recommended or a quart per every 1000 calories of intake. More is needed if you exercise briskly or live in a hot environment.

Most of our body is composed of water. Maintaining hydration helps our thought processes, increases fat metabolism, reduces water retention, increases our energy levels, and improves our organ function. Spread your intake throughout the day. Do not count caffeinated beverages. Drink additional water to cover this.

You need to eat! Eating raises your metabolism. Think "eat and burn". You should have six meals a day that are balanced within the proportions above. Nutrition for athletes, men and women should differ only slightly.

Watch your sodium. Your total daily sodium intake should not exceed 2400 mg/day.

Eating to reduce fat composition

As we discussed earlier, many of us are watching what we eat to lose body fat. With this regard, there are some concerns in addition to balancing our nutrients:

Portion Control. As we mentioned, one of the big reasons we are overfat is because we eat too much of the wrong things. Even when you have adjusted your proportions of carbs, proteins and fats, you can still have too much of a good thing.

The general rule is to “eat when you are hungry and stop eating when you are satisfied”. This is a simple, natural rule that truly works when executed properly. Execution is the complicated part.

The “eat when you are hungry” portion of the equation is difficult, as most of us are constrained with time limits due to work and other obligations. Because you are supposed to wait until you are hungry, when you eat will also be affected by how much you eat at each meal. Then there is the whole question of what hunger feels like and how hungry should I be before I eat?.

Then there is the “stop when you are satisfied” part. Most of us have heard that it takes 20 minutes after a meal to realize we are satisfied. Eat a little, wait 20 minutes... eat a little more, wait 20 minutes? Not very practical.

Simple rule. Complicated application.

Most credible sources recommend 5-6 smaller meals per day rather than the 2-3 larger ones. You’ll want to size each of these meals so you are hungry for the next one. If you have forgotten what hunger really feels like, don’t eat for a while. Let your stomach churn and burn a bit to remind you of how you were designed to desire food.

Estimating Calorie Intake. Along with portion control, one way to determine approximately how much you should eat is by estimating calorie intake. To estimate the amount of calories you need in a day, multiply your body weight by the following factors, considering lifestyle:

Sedentary lifestyle (no aerobic exercise):
Males: 12, Females – 10

Moderately Active (aerobic exercise 3 times/week):
Males: 15, Females 13

Active (aerobic exercise 5 times/week):
Males 17, Females: 15

This will give you an estimated starting point of calorie intake to maintain your current weight. For instance, if you are an active female, weighing 140 pounds, you need an estimated:140 X 15 = 2100 calories per day to maintain your weight.

If you want to lose weight, you can figure it will take 3500 calories to "burn" a pound of fat. So to lose a pound in a week, we would need to reduce calorie intake by 3500 ÷ 7 = 500 calories per day. For the example above, the women would need to an approximate intake of 2100 – 500 = 1600 calories per day to lose a pound in one week. Generally, you should not go below 1200 –1500 calories per day, or your metabolic rate will drop.

Helpful hints

- The first steps are to make some simple changes to what you already eat. There's a good chance you are eating right most of the time. It may just be that handful of M&M's in the afternoon that causes your energy level to peak and dive that is causing you difficulty. So focus on simple changes. Don't deviate initially too much from things you like unless they are really bad for you (smoking, eating quantities of donuts, cakes, and cookies regularly). If you do, it will decrease your odds of sticking with the program.
- Cheat one day a week or once in a while. It helps psychologically and physically. Eat the things you like and crave.
- If you "lose it" for a day, don't worry about it. Get back in the saddle the next day and try again.
- Watch putting all your focus on eating healthy foods and not keeping balance in mind. Vegetables, fruits, vitamins, herbs, etc. are all components of a healthy diet, but are not exclusive. You need protein and fat in your diet.
- Take part in pleasurable activities that aren't related to food.
- Turn meal times into special focused breaks from the daily routine.
- Avoid eating while watching TV or reading.
- Chew slowly to fully enjoy meals.
- Learn the pleasures of shopping for healthy foods. Good food, exercise and a positive attitude really help people reach and maintain a healthy weight, and that creates a strong sense of accomplishment and personal satisfaction.

- Many of the packaged, frozen meals (Lean Cuisine, Healthy Choice) have the correct proportions of carbs, protein, and fat. Having them a couple of times a week may help save time in preparation. These are, however, processed foods typically with a lot of salt. Feel free to add more fresh vegetables to round out the meal.

Summary – Chapter Six

- Eat for good health. Restrictive diets do not work long-term. Estimate your calorie intake and don't starve yourself. Do not go below 1400 calories per day.
- Don't deviate initially too much from things you like. Work to reduce your intake of refined, processed foods, simple sugars, saturated fats, and alcohol. These have minimal, if any, nutritional value and the extra calories get stored as fat. If you do, it will decrease your odds of sticking with the program. Take small steps in changing your eating habits.
- Six smaller meals per day are better than three to maintain energy levels and for losing body fat. Include protein, carbohydrate, and fat in each.
- Drink at least 8-10 cups of water per day. (one quart per 1000 calories of food intake).
- Cheat one day a week or once in a while. It helps.
- Balance carbohydrates, proteins and fats. Recommended per RDA: 55-60% of your calorie intake is to be Carbohydrates, less than 30% Fat and 15-20% Protein. There are 9 calories/gram of fat and 4 calories/gram of carbohydrates and protein. Balance out each of your meals within the percentages listed.
- The Food Guide Pyramid is the most reputable guide going to show portions of each food group that should be consumed.
- Watch your portions. Read the container and measure

out initially until you get a good idea what you should be eating. Use your hunger to guide you to when you should eat. Stop eating when you are satisfied.

- Look to fresh, whole grained sources as well as fresh fruits and vegetables for your source of carbohydrates.
- Eat within 1-2 hours before a workout for fuel and within 1-2 hours after for recovery.
- Fat is important, but should limited. If you are overweight, cut your fat to 20% and increase protein intake to 20% for faster weight loss. Saturated fat intake should be below 10% to help control cholesterol. Desirable cholesterol: less than 200 mg/dl.
- Protein intake should not exceed 30% of the calories in your diet. This is unhealthy. Minimum is 12%.
- Sugar intake should be moderated, particularly if you are overweight. Refined sugar, as the primary ingredient of a snack or meal will affect your energy levels.
- Animal proteins are the best source for all the amino acids necessary to build muscle and tissue. Lean proteins from chicken and fish are preferred. Egg whites are also an excellent source.
- At least two servings of dairy products per day are essential. More for perimenopause and menopausal women.
- Vitamins and minerals are essential nutrients. A multivitamin is a good idea, though if you are eating with balance, you won't need to supplement. Vitamins C and E and calcium are advised.
- Meal supplements, though not necessary, may help balance out meals easier and will help when you don't have time to cook. Look for products within the calorie percentages above. Avoid high protein bars and weight gain products.
- Nutrition for athletes, men, and women should differ

only slightly.

- Sodium intake should not exceed 2400 mg/day.
- 20-30g of dietary fiber per day is recommended.

Chapter 7

Aerobic Exercise

It's too bad we have to exercise; but we do.

This may seem odd coming from someone who has owned a small health club for the past 16 years, but the truth of the matter is that we must exercise in order to replace the lack of activity in our lives. We are less active than ever and as a result are experiencing health problems.

The CDC's report on Physical Activity and Health notes that up until the 20th century, people performed most of their physical activity as part of their occupations. In Western populations, occupation related physical demands have declined and the availability of leisure time has grown. In the past 30 years, technological advancements in automation have taken even more physical work out of our lives.

Though we have less activity in our working lives, public awareness of the benefits of exercise has resulted in people spending more of their leisure time being physically active. We attempt to compensate for the lack of activity in our working lives by supplementing with exercise in our off-time. In nature, mammals are active while searching for food or during play; humans are not much different. If there is limited activity in "making a living", then the activity outlet must be during "play time".

In our search for leisure activities that will help us develop and maintain our physical well-being, we need to find those that develop our cardiovascular system as well as strengthen our muscles and bones. Many sports related activities such as basketball and golf may do well for cardiovascular conditioning, but the regularity with which these activities can be done is not generally frequent enough to keep us in shape.

To make up for an inactive work life, a substantial amount of activity during our leisure time must be inserted.

We exercise to replace the activity we no longer have in our lives. We jog on the treadmill for 30 minutes per day to replace the many miles we used to walk before the automobile. We lift weights to replace the tasks of carrying food and water, chopping wood, etc. Our exercise program should develop our bodies completely as they are designed to be used. Because we don't have a lot of extra time, we also want an efficient exercise regiment that gets results without wasted time.

The Center for Disease Control recommends "a minimum of 30 minutes of physical activity of moderate intensity (such as brisk walking) on most, if not all, days of the week. It is also acknowledged that for most people, greater health benefits can be obtained by engaging in physical activity of more vigorous intensity or of longer duration."

This is our goal for America.

But before we go hog-wild on our cardio routine, there are some considerations. First and foremost, you have to make sure your body is up to it. Check with your doctor. Make sure you're not doing too much, too fast.

Aerobic Activity

The term "aerobic" means "to use oxygen". This is what aerobic activities do – get your lungs working and your heart pumping. Examples of aerobic activities are walking, jogging, biking, swimming, etc. Doing aerobic exercise should not be confused with aerobic dance or simply "aerobics". Though aerobic dance is certainly aerobic, when we are referring to aerobic activity, we are talking about any activity that gets your heart pumping.

Aerobic activities strengthen the heart and cardiovascular system. They will also help burn calories and help lose fat over our entire body. This helps us see muscle definition underneath. Because there is no way to spot reduce fat, like in the abdominal area, aerobic activity helps reduce overall body fat, which will keep us trim all over.

What is considered "moderate intensity"?

Per the CDC guidelines, we want 30 minutes of aerobic activity of *moderate intensity* most days of the week. Moderate intensity can be defined as any activity that gets your heart pumping between 60% and 80% of its maximum. This level of intensity is considered beneficial for cardiovascular health. You can estimate your maximum heart rate by subtracting your age from 220.

Your target heart rate zone (THZ) is defined as being between 60% and 80% of this maximum. This is where you want your heart rate for maximum benefit.

For a 40 year old man:

Maximum = 220 – 40 (age) = 180

THZ (lower limit) = 180 X .6 = 108 beats per minute

THZ (upper limit) = 180 X .8 = 144 bpm

When exercising, take your pulse for 10 seconds, then multiply by 6.

If our 40 year-old man measures 28 beats in 10 seconds, his heart rate would be:

28 X 6 = 168 bpm

Slow down Hercules! You're 24 bpm above target.

If you start to get serious about training and particularly if you are high risk, try a heart rate monitor. The best kind (considering expense and accuracy) are the ones with a chest strap. There is no guessing or stopping to measure your pulse. You can get features on them to let you know when you are out of your zone as well.

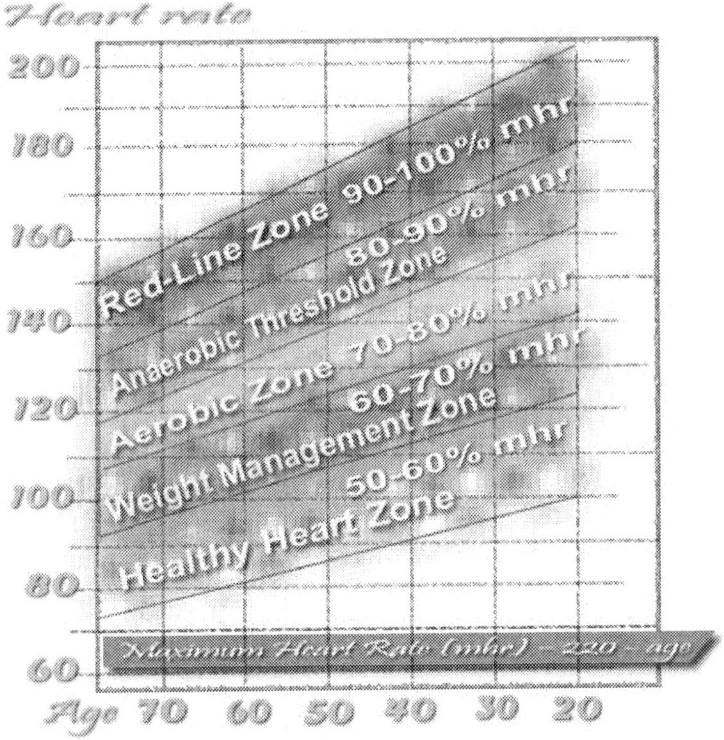

Getting Started

Your first few minutes of exercise will be your "warm-up". Start slow and work up to your THZ over 5 minutes. This will reduce your chance of injury. As you exercise, you'll want to monitor your intensity by checking your THZ.

As mentioned in Chapter 4, monitor how you feel during your exercise. Base your effort on a scale of 1-10. Aim for an effort of 7. This will usually mean you are in the zone. At this point it's like you are late for an appointment and can talk in short sentences with concentrated effort. Your breathing increases as your oxygen need increases. As your level of fitness increases, you will be able to stay at this level longer. To "cool down" slow your activity down to decrease your heart rate back to pre-exercise levels. This takes a few minutes also, and is very important for your heart to recover. The less time it takes your heart rate to recover, the healthier it is. Also in Chapter 4, we discussed RHR as a means to measure your heart's efficiency. Before you get out of bed in the morning, take your pulse for a full minute. As you become more fit, your RHR will decrease.

Walking briskly is the universal exercise recommended for beginners, whether on a treadmill or outdoors. If walking doesn't work for you, biking might be an option. Keep an eye on your heart rate, though. Leisurely riding may not get you where you need to be. Another option that is less strenuous on joints than either biking or walking is working on an elliptical trainer. These new machines work well for some people with back or knee problems. This should be evaluated on an individual basis, however.

Although the recommended aerobic duration is 30 minutes, 5 times a week, 20 minutes, 3 times per week is considered beneficial for your heart. You may want to increase or decrease the amount of aerobic activity from what is recommended based on your lifestyle (sedentary vs. active) or your goals. If walking is an exercise you love to do, then certainly don't limit yourself to 30 minutes. How do you know when you are doing too much? Your body will tell you. If you ache and are tired all the time and you're walking 6 miles per day, chances are you are over-training.

Over-training is not just a function of too much training. It is also a function of what you eat and how much recovery time you have. Remember; your goal is to feel great. If you are overdoing it, it will work to the contrary.

Interval Training

Interval training, where you increase and decrease intensity during the workout, can shorten your routine substantially and burn more calories. If you are on a limited time budget, interval training gets the job done in short order. It is also a great means of altering your workout.

Here's a typical interval training routine: Take any exercise you do, walking, running, biking, etc., and change the intensity as follows:

- 2 minutes low intensity – 60% THZ
- 2 minutes medium intensity – 70% THZ
- 1-2 minutes higher intensity – 80% THZ
- Repeat cycle 3-4 times
- End with 2-minute low intensity cool down, for a total of 17-26 minutes.

Try this 2-3 times a week and you'll be surprised by the results. Interval training should be tried after you are accustomed to exercise and may not be suited for beginners.

Change your routine

Varying your aerobic routine prevents your body from adaptation and hitting a plateau where improvement is stifled. For instance, if you are jogging and your speed does not improve or you don't seem to be able to go as far as you would like, it may be time to change to something else.

Changes in your aerobic routine include changing the intensity, duration and/or changing the type. Try biking a couple days per week to give your joints a rest. If you walk briskly 5 days per week for 30 minutes, then try walking 45 minutes one day.

But whatever you do, don't overdo the aerobic portion of

your program. You might think if 30 minutes of exercise is good, 45 minutes is better. How much you should do depends on your level of fitness and your goals. For instance, if you are trying to lose fat, it is advised to accumulate 45-60 minutes of aerobic activity most days of the week. But don't just do aerobic activity. Balance your program with strength training and flexibility exercises.

Ask your trainer. Your personal trainer will help you plan your aerobic exercise routine based on your goals. She will know how to develop a safe aerobic exercise based on your current level of fitness. A program will be designed to incorporate your target heart rate and duration of exercise.

No substitute for laziness

Even those of us that do our aerobic exercise religiously still spend considerable time and effort trying to find the closest parking spot at the local Walmart to spare ourselves the walk.

As you know now, it is the lack of activity in our lives that causes many of the health problems we have. Exercise is a substitute for this activity. If we had the activity, we would not need the exercise. So why work so hard to save a few extra steps?

- Take the stairs instead of the elevator.
- Pick a remote parking spot that will give you a few extra steps.
- Walk to the Post Office, bank, etc., for errands if they're within a mile of where you live. Buy the necessary clothing to travel in foul weather. If you live farther than a mile, buy a basket or carrying rack for your bike.
- Feel a little goofy carrying a tote bag around? Keep in mind that it's this "goofy" feeling that keeps many of us where we are today.

Get up and get going!

Walking – A Good Way to Start Your Program

Walking is one of the simplest, most natural forms of exercise. In many ways, walking is an ideal exercise. It requires no special equipment or knowledge and can be done almost anywhere. Injuries are rare in walkers who train at a reasonable pace and wear well-fitted walking shoes. Walking is a low-impact activity that is well-suited to those that are trying to lose weight and condition their cardiovascular system. Walking is also considered a weight-bearing exercise which helps prevent osteoporosis. Depending on your goals, your walking program can be adapted.

For cardiovascular health, you will need to walk briskly enough to get your heart rate in your THZ. Changing stride lengths, increasing the pace, and swinging your arms broadly at your sides all increase the intensity of the activity. You can also increase intensity by walking up hills or using walking poles like in cross-country skiing. For weight reduction or for those that have been inactive for a long time, a slower pace and a longer duration may be recommended.

Walkers should exercise three to five days a week for 20 to 45 minutes each time. If you walk a lot through the day, you can also use a pedometer to count your steps accumulated.

Rules for Pain-Free Walking

To prevent walking injuries, follow these guidelines:

- Exercise good posture and heel-to-toe motion.
- Warm up gradually to a brisk walking pace.
- Avoid sudden increases in distance and walking speed.
- The only special equipment a fitness walker needs is a comfortable pair of shoes. Wear walking shoes with thick soles and cushioned insoles.
- Walk on soft, smooth surfaces whenever possible.

- Wear two pairs of socks if blisters are a problem.
- As with all aerobic activity, vigorous walking needs a warm-up and cool-down period.

Walking Injuries

Walking at a casual pace usually presents no problems, but race-walking or "exercise-walking" to increase the aerobic benefit may increase the risk of injury. Injuries that walkers might experience include:

- shin splints, with pain in the muscles of the front of the lower leg;
- muscle cramps, or charley horses;
- Achilles tendonitis, with pain especially in the ankle and back of the lower leg;
- foot injuries, such as a bruised heel or blisters.

The Best Treatment

Most soft tissue injuries respond to the treatment known by the acronym RICE:

- **R**est: Avoid activity until the affected area is healed and then return to activity gradually.
- **I**ce: Put an ice pack on the affected area for about 20 minutes three or four times a day, taking care not to freeze the skin.
- **C**ompression: Use an elastic bandage around the affected area or tape around a foot, taking care not to cut off circulation.
- **E**levation: Keep the injured area above the heart. When lying down, for instance, an injured leg can rest on pillows.
- A muscle cramp can be massaged and soaked in warm water until it relaxes. Persistent foot injuries will require an examination by a health care provider.

Summary – Chapter Seven

- Check with your physician prior to starting any routine.
- If you don't know already, learn about your target heart rate zone. Recommendation: buy a heart rate monitor.
- Exercising 30 minutes five days per week in your target heart rate zone is the goal. 20 minutes every other day will also benefit.
- Changing the type of aerobic activity prevents your body from adaptation and hitting a plateau where improvement is stifled.
- One or two 45-minute aerobic sessions per week are also beneficial.
- Interval training (changing intensity during your aerobic exercise) is effective and can save time.

Chapter 8

Strength Training

Strength training should be an integral part of everyone's exercise routine. The term strength training encompasses both resistance training and the more specific weight training. *Resistance training* refers to the use of resistance to develop strength and/or muscle size. This includes training with weights (gravity), resistance bands, etc. Weight training is specific to using weights (gravity) to build strength and muscle.

Some people are reluctant to try strength training for fear of developing the large bulky muscles of bodybuilders. The training required to develop the muscle mass of a bodybuilder is very different than a program designed for an average person. Most body builders lift 2-3 hours everyday and are usually genetically endowed. The average person only needs to lift 2-3 hours per week to maintain healthy, strong muscles. Women particularly need not worry about 'bulking up' from strength training, as they only have a fraction of the testosterone hormone that men have, which is responsible for building massive muscles.

Essential to a "well rounded" exercise program.

In the 1950's, strength training with weights was solely practiced by those who were involved with sports such as bodybuilding or weight lifting. In the years that followed, strength training became more popular with young men involved with athletics or concerned with having a muscular physique. Today, as all the benefits of weight training are being discovered, fitness experts are recommending weight training as part of a "well rounded" exercise program for both men and women of any age.

Strength Training Benefits

Strength training puts strength activity back into our lives. Many Americans in their thirties, especially women, are not active enough and start losing muscle tissue and strength. Although this decline in strength is sometimes associated with aging, it is more likely linked to inactivity. Strength training builds the muscle tissue thereby maintaining our strength.

Strength Training effects how you feel about yourself. Strength training along with a balanced diet, proper rest and aerobic exercise make for a healthy lifestyle and directly effects how you feel about yourself. People who are fit feel better and as a result are more confident and have higher self-esteem. They do not feel winded when they climb stairs or shovel snow. They do not groan when carrying in grocery bags. Those who take the time to exercise are concerned about self - and as a result feel better about themselves.

Strength training can increase your stamina and decrease the stiffness felt from inactivity. It can strengthen the back so to alleviate pain often associated with weak lower back muscles. A strong back supports a better posture, which gives you a confident appearance. Because weak muscles are often responsible for many injuries, strength training also acts as a preventative measure. The self-confidence built from being strong is something that is difficult to describe and should be experienced.

Strength Training helps with weight control. You have probably heard statistics quoted that claim "diets do not work for weight loss". It is fact that the majority of 'dieters' return to their old ways and are seldom successful.

One study conducted at Houston's Baylor College of Medicine tested this hypothesis on 165 men and women who were at least 30 pounds overweight. They evaluated subjects after

12 subsequent, unsupervised months: Members of a diet-only group had regained all the lost weight and were an average 2 pounds heavier than when they started. The diet plus exercise group had regained 14.7 pounds, leaving them 4.9 pounds lighter than when they started. The exercise only group, however, leveled off and maintained its loss of 6.4 pounds.

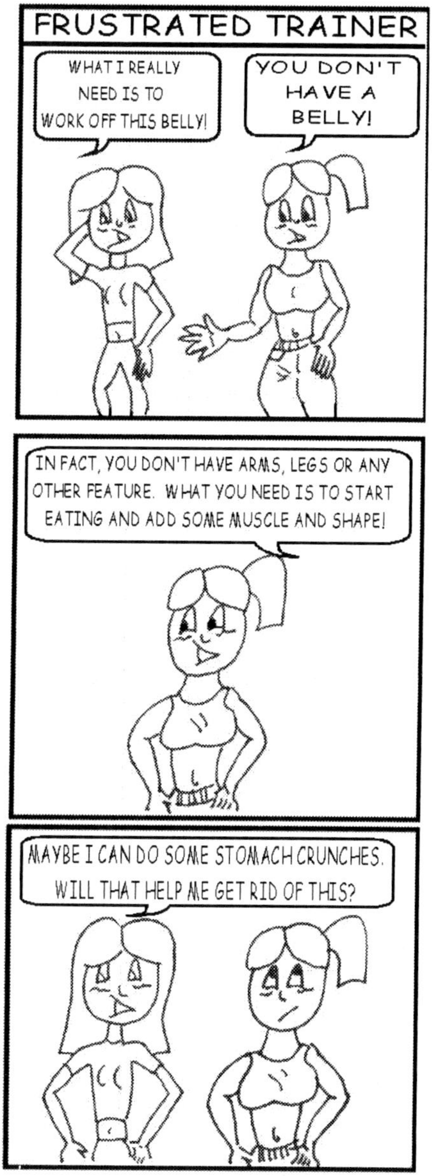

FRUSTRATED TRAINER
WHAT I REALLY NEED IS TO WORK OFF THIS BELLY!
YOU DON'T HAVE A BELLY!
IN FACT, YOU DON'T HAVE ARMS, LEGS OR ANY OTHER FEATURE. WHAT YOU NEED IS TO START EATING AND ADD SOME MUSCLE AND SHAPE!
MAYBE I CAN DO SOME STOMACH CRUNCHES. WILL THAT HELP ME GET RID OF THIS?

One can conclude from this study, along with many more, that exercise is important for weight control.

So if you exercise, you can eat anything you want and not be fat, right? No. Remember that fitness is the result of proper diet, adequate rest and exercise. Your body requires a **balanced** diet along with exercise. Eating right in conjunction with exercise or activity is the best way to lose fat, and more importantly, maintain a healthy body composition.

When you strength train, keep in mind there is no such thing as turning fat into muscle of vice versa. A better way to look at it is that fat can be reduced and muscle tissue can be built. To reduce fat, one can 1) increase the rate at which calories (supplied by food) are burned and/or 2) reduce the intake of calories and fat. Many people concerned with losing weight are interested in the number of calories burned during exercise. In a typical session, aerobic exercise burns substantially more calories than anaerobic exercise. This is because the body's metabolism - the way it breaks down and uses food - is increased temporarily during the workout. But what about after the workout?

It takes more calories per pound for your body to maintain muscle tissue than fat tissue. Just like a more powerful engine needs more gas, a strong body needs fuel (high performance, preferably) to keep it going. It has been estimated that it takes up to 60 calories to maintain a pound of muscle per day. Compare this to the 2-3 calories per day required to maintain a pound of fat. <u>Metabolism is subsequently increased when muscle tissue is developed</u>. Weight training is much more effective at building muscle than aerobic exercise; hence it is more effective at raising metabolic rate before and after the workout. This increased metabolic rate offers lasting benefits to a weight reduction program.

<u>It prevents osteoporosis and strengthens bones.</u> Osteoporosis is a bone-thinning disease that tends to strike women after menopause, though men can develop it as well. Weight bearing exercise negates the effect of the disease. Walking has been proven to decrease the rate at which bone density is lost, but only strength training has been proven to actually increase bone density. The stress put on bones by strength training results in an increase in bone density. Because osteoporosis decreases bone mass and can result in an

increased risk of bone fractures, strength training is especially important to women.

It gives you what you are looking for. Aerobic exercise - walking, jogging, biking etc. - is of primary importance for good health. As discussed, it conditions the heart and the respiratory system and builds stamina. It "adds years to your life and life to your years". Aerobic exercise *should be* the main concern for everyone as it is most important for good health. But developing CRE and longevity are not the only reasons for which people exercise. Many people are looking to 'tone-up'. Weight training is more effective at shaping and toning upper body muscles than walking, jogging or biking. Those who are looking to 'tone-up' and improve posture get the results they are looking for with weight training more so than they would with aerobic exercise. This is another reason why strength training and aerobic exercise should go hand in hand in an exercise routine.

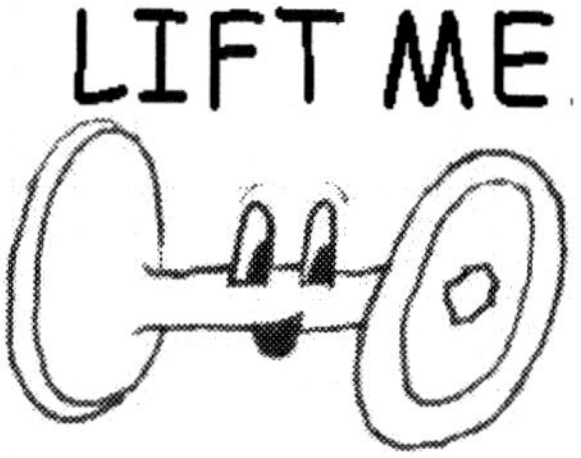

How it works

Once your aerobic exercise is a habit, it is time to add strength training to your program. Before you start, it is important that you understand the mechanics behind it so you can optimize the results from your training without risking injury.

The human body has fascinating ways of adapting for different 'loads' or stresses put on it by its environment. Muscle development is achieved by using the body's natural adaptation mechanisms. If the body finds itself in a situation where increased strength or stamina is required, it will adapt - over time - to handle the load. If you have ever started a job which required you to do hard work you have never done before, you know this to be true. For the first few days, you might be real sore, but once you have been doing it a while, it becomes much easier.

Strength training uses the body's natural adaptations for conditioning. By loading body parts through strength training, muscles will grow to accommodate the demands made on it.

Personal Trainers teach proper training techniques and design safe, effective strength training programs. It is essential to get instruction in proper use of training equipment. Your trainer will create and individual, progressive program for you. The following sequence gives general guidelines and will help reinforce what your trainer will tell you, however, it is no substitute for the knowledge your trainer will offer.

Rules for Safe, Effective Weight Training

<u>Rule #1 - Always warm up</u>. The muscles, tendons and ligaments need blood to function properly. Prior to working out, five to ten minutes of aerobic exercise and a light static stretch will give the muscles the needed oxygen to perform. Warm ups reduce chance of injury and improve the performance of the muscles, which will optimize the results you will get. A good walk and stretch will do the job.

<u>Rule #2 - Always cool down</u>. A static stretch of the muscles worked at the end of your routine will increase blood flow and reduce soreness.

<u>Rule #3 - All movements are to be slow and controlled</u>. Slow, controlled movements obtain the best results from strength training. Quick, explosive movements tend to work the muscles involved in the beginning of the movement harder than through the rest of the movement. Think slow

movements for fast results.

Rule #4 - Breathe continuously. Improper breathing techniques can cause the blood pressure to rise. It may seem natural to hold your breath during a strenuous movement, but don't. Exhale during the strained part of the exercise (Exhale, Exert) and inhale during the easier portion of the movement.

Rule #5 - Use a full range of motion. To develop the muscle group you are working properly, use a full range of motion in doing the exercise.

Rule #6 - Monitor closely the time you rest between sets of exercises. The general rule is to wait one minute between sets of the same exercise. Not waiting long enough or waiting too long between sets of the same exercise will not optimize muscle development. Note: Waiting between exercises that work different muscle groups is not necessary.

Rule #7 - Sufficient recovery time between workouts. In general, working the same muscles everyday is not a good idea. A day or two of recovery in between workouts will give the best results. Strength training actually breaks down muscle tissue. Gains in strength occur as the muscle rebuilds between workouts.

Remember: Diet and rest are key players in optimizing the results obtained from strength training. Keep an eye on the whole for best overall results.

Intensity

Intensity refers to the amount of effort put into an exercise. Having the right level of intensity is key to results. Insufficient intensity will minimize results; however, excessive intensity can lead to over-training which could also reduce results. Worse yet, too much intensity can lead to injury.

Beginners need to develop a feel for proper intensity. Here

are some guidelines:

- The last repetition of an exercise should be challenging. It should be difficult, but never to the point of compromising form. Let's take biceps curls for example. If you are to do 10 repetitions of the exercise, the tenth one should be difficult, but not to the point that you use other muscles, such as your back, to help. Maintaining good form is most important. If the last rep is not difficult, add more weight.
- If you find that your muscles are very sore the next day, you might want to back off on either the number of sets, the number of exercises or the intensity. A certain amount of discomfort following a workout is expected. However, not being able to move means you probably went overboard.

Getting Started

Step One - Check with your physician

As with any exercise program, it is always a good idea to discuss it with your doctor before diving in, especially if you:

1) are over 30 and have not exercised in over 3 years
2) have any health problems that could be adversely affected by lifting.

Strength training puts stress on the joints, muscles and heart. Your doctor's blessing should be foremost in starting to exercise.

Step two - Develop an aerobic routine

The next important step is to fit an exercise routine into your schedule. If you do not already have a regular aerobic exercise routine, such as walking, this should be the first step. Make the time in your schedule to exercise.

Step Three - Learn the proper way to workout

There are two concerns in learning to exercise: doing exercises that promote injury and doing exercises incorrectly.

Many of the exercises done 20 years ago are now considered harmful, particularly those exercises which over stress the joints and back. Examples are deep knee bends and sit-ups. Other exercises may be harmful to some but not to others. People who are in excellent physical condition may isolate certain muscle groups by doing certain exercise movements. For the beginner, this would not be appropriate, as isolation exercises can over-stress the muscles.

Exercising properly is necessary for safety and for maximum muscle development. Doing it the right way involves...

1) exerting the right amount of effort.
2) using proper technique/form
3) having the correct number of repetitions/sets
4) using the correct weight.
5) proper warm-up and cool-down exercises

Refer to the workout guidelines attached. Strength training the right way should be foremost in your workout to avoid injury and maximize results.

Terminology

Repetitions (Reps)- The number of times an exercise movement is performed

Sets - A group of repetitions of an exercise movement followed by an interval of rest

Failure - The point at which the muscle can no longer do the movement.

The Regimen

The beginning exercise regimen should include:

1) 8-12 'basic' exercises which train all body parts
2) 1-2 sets of 8-12 repetitions for each exercise. Beginners

may start with one set and work up to 3.

3) 2-3 sessions per week with at least a day of rest in between sessions.

A typical session should last about 30-45 minutes. If you find you are excessively sore or tired with the above routine, try adjusting the intensity of the workout and build up to where the routine does not cause overexertion. Adjusting the intensity can be done by 1) allowing shorter or longer breaks between sets and exercises 2) increasing/decreasing the weight or 3) increasing/decreasing the number of repetitions. If you find you are not getting results in your routine, chances are you are not working hard or long enough. Try increasing intensity, repetitions or number of exercises. Not getting results may also be a sign of a stagnated routine. Try changing or adding new exercises.

Selecting the 'right' weight

Ideally, the last repetition in a set of exercises should be at or near failure. Those in poor physical condition may not push their bodies to this point, but for those who are conditioned, this is the goal. With this in mind, the right weight would be that which brought the muscles to failure in the last repetition of the set. If the last reps were too easy, then the logical step would be to increase the weight and vice versa. This is an example of how weight training is individualized.

Of course, the ideal is not always possible or practical. Weights are available in certain increments, so the ideal weight may not be available. Also, the last set of exercises probably will have fewer reps than the first, as the muscles are fatigued. Perhaps the first set will consist of 11 reps where as the third will have only 9. Experience and proper training will make workout weight decisions easier.

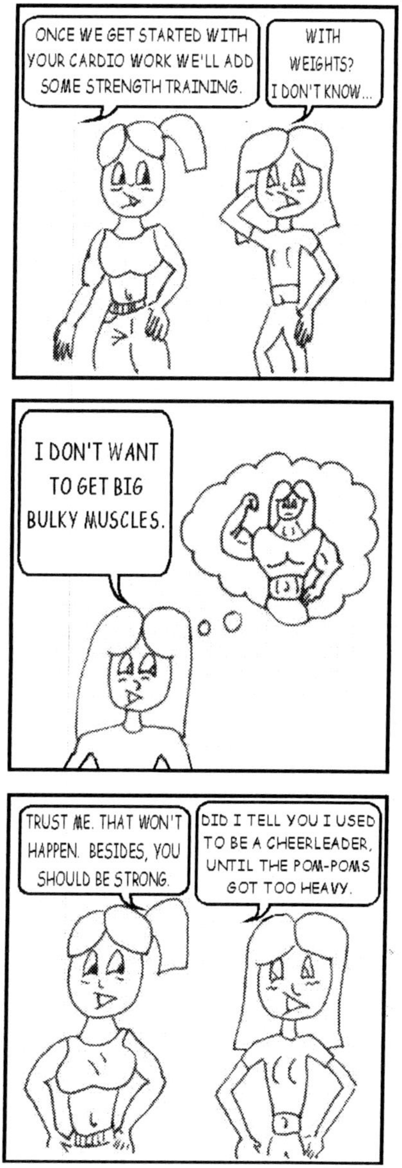
ONCE WE GET STARTED WITH YOUR CARDIO WORK WE'LL ADD SOME STRENGTH TRAINING.
WITH WEIGHTS? I DON'T KNOW...
I DON'T WANT TO GET BIG BULKY MUSCLES.
TRUST ME. THAT WON'T HAPPEN. BESIDES, YOU SHOULD BE STRONG.
DID I TELL YOU I USED TO BE A CHEERLEADER, UNTIL THE POM-POMS GOT TOO HEAVY.

Staying Motivated

As indicated, there are a host of good reasons for everyone to strength train, namely to improve health and appearance. Some people start lifting weights with a short-term goal in mind like shaping up after having a baby or before going on a cruise. This is fine, but if you decide you want to make weight training a part of your life, it will require constant motivation.

Your trainer is the best tool you can employ to keep your motivation up. This is one of the primary reasons to hire a trainer: to keep you moving through the good and not-so-good times.

The best motivation for continuing training is results. As you start feeling better and see improvement, you will be driven to continue. If you consistently weight train 2-3 times a week, you should see and feel visible changes after one month. Perhaps not a loss of weight, but a shift in muscle/fat ratio. Your muscles will be stronger, firmer and shapelier. You may notice your clothes fitting better and some loss of inches. You may also realize what a great stress reducer weight training is and how you gained a more positive outlook.

As you continue to train, however, the results may not be so evident. Just because it is less visually apparent does not mean you are not still getting results. This is why it is necessary to keep an accurate record of your progression. You should record the weight you workout with along with the number of reps and sets. Also, keep track of all your measurements and weight, at least on a monthly basis. This way even if your results are not visible to the eye, you will still 'see' improvement. Record your results. You may also want to include a food diary or other fitness related records in the notebook as well. It is not important how you do it only that you do it.

Another hint to staying motivated is to make an effort to workout even if you have a long day. You will be surprised how your attitude will change once you workout.

A third way to stay motivated would be to take on a workout partner on those days you are not working with a trainer. A partner will push you on the days you do not feel like exercising, as you will push her when she does not feel up to it. Having someone to workout with also makes it more fun and if you enjoy what you are doing you are more apt to stick with it.

Ready?... Then let's get started!

Now that you know the benefits of strength training and have some ideas on how it should be done, it is time to go to work. The most difficult step is the first one - to start. It is difficult because even though you may have thrown out all the misconceptions about weight training, you still may not be sure if it is right for you.

Well, there is only one way to find out!

Commit to sticking to your trainer's program for at least 12 weeks. You need to give it at least this long for a fair test. After you give it a fair shot, you will agree that strength training should be part of **everyone'**s fitness routine.

Summary – Chapter 8

- Strength Training is essential to <u>everyone</u> for strong muscles and bones.
- Learn how to do it safely and effectively. Proper form is first priority.
- Allow sufficient recovery time between workouts.
- Fancy equipment is not necessary. A couple of pairs of dumbbells and a bench are all that is needed.
- Try a fit-ball or exercise bands – they're simple, inexpensive pieces of equipment that get results.

Tips for Safe Exercise

As stated, one of your objectives for your program should be and injury-free exercise regimen. Follow these simple points and minimize your chances of getting hurt.

Warm Up and Cool Down

The most important times for preventing fitness injuries is during the critical periods before and after exercise. Warming up for five minutes prior to vigorous exercise with gentle aerobic activities, such as a walk, will increase the blood flow to inactive muscles. Gradually raise your heart rate to its target zone without shock. Do the same when you are finishing your workout. Bring your heart rate down gradually by decreasing intensity (slowing down) for 5 minutes.

Gentle static stretching should be part of the warm up and cool down process. Stretching before exercise loosens tight muscles and improves joint flexibility. This reduces your risk of sprains and strains. Concentrate on stretching those muscle groups used in your particular activity. For example, runners will want to concentrate on stretching out the legs, while swimmers will want to pay extra attention to upper body muscles. Static stretching for a few minutes after exercise is also recommended to prevent muscle soreness and to improve your overall level of flexibility.

Don't Push Too Hard

More important than not working hard enough is working too hard. For aerobic activity, track your heart rate. A heart rate monitor is a good investment, as it will help keep you in your training zone. With strength training, select the proper resistance for the exercise and don't push until the veins pop out of your head!

Select the right equipment to exercise.

Properly suited and fitted running shoes are important for walkers and runners alike. Make sure you take the time and spend the money to get you something that does not hurt you during the activity.

With all the choices of exercise equipment today, you should be able to find one that is comfortable and does not aggravate joints or past injuries. Elliptical trainers are high intensity, yet low-impact machines that are proven to help certain people with joint problems. Recumbent bicycles not only take your weight off of your limbs, they also support your back and are easy to get on and off of. Pick the equipment that makes you the most comfortable.

Bicycling is an excellent outdoor activity, if the bike is properly fitted for you. Don't let the bike store talk you into handlebars that are uncomfortable, just because they're the style these days. Make sure your seat is set properly and you have all the necessary safety equipment. An ill-fitting bicycle can lead to back and knee pain or injury. Make sure that your equipment is in top condition before risking your health and safety.

Use common sense and be safe

Use all necessary safety equipment and if you are exercising out in the sun, don't forget your sunscreen. If you are walking and running on roads with traffic, always face the proper direction – facing traffic. If you are biking on main roads, always bike on the side of the road going with the traffic and stay off the sidewalks. If you're traveling in unfamiliar territory, go slow enough to see all the ruts and potholes in plenty of time to avoid them.

Safety gear may make you feel awkward the first few times you wear it, but keep in mind the inconvenience of wearing the gear is outweighed by the safety benefits. Select gear that you like and that fits well to eliminate or minimize the awkwardness.

Using common sense when exercising and be patient when starting your program. Keep in mind you'll be doing this for a long time and though you may be anxious to get going, don't let your drive cause you to do something foolish. Take the time to do it right with injury-free exercise as the objective.

Chapter 9

Flexibility and Stretching

As we pointed out, flexibility - the freedom to bend your joints and stretch your muscles in any normal direction without stiffness or resistance - is a very important element of total fitness. It is also one of the least promoted. In most fitness books, including this one, it is included only after everything else!

Stretching

Gentle static stretching exercises are perhaps the best means of keeping your muscles and joints flexible. Recent studies are showing that the timing of stretching is not as important as once thought. Stretching before exercise does not prevent muscle pulls. However, stretching is important and can be done at any point in your exercise routine, as well as on rest days. Stretching is <u>the</u> way to improve flexibility.

The best way to stretch a muscle is to do it slowly and gently. When you reach your maximum pain-free stretch, don't bounce. Just hold the stretch until your muscle relaxes, usually 10 to 20 seconds. Because of this holding period, these types of stretches are called "static" stretches. Static stretches safely elongate your muscles as well as the tendons that attach them to the bone, thereby improving joint mobility.

The benefits of stretching are:

- Improved joint mobility. Flexible muscles allow your joints to move freely.
- Improved performance during activity. Stretching increases the blood flow to the muscles and the joints.

- Reduced risk of injury. Flexible joints and muscles are less likely to get injured when you have to lift, catch, or move something, or when you exercise or lift weights. Properly warmed up and stretched, your muscles, tendons and ligaments are less likely to fail you during activity.
- Decreased joint aches and pains. If you ache every morning when you get up, it could be the result of insufficient stretching.

Some important points about stretching:

- AS mentioned, the best way to improve your flexibility is a program of gentle stretching.
- Do not bounce or jerk when you stretch. Fight the urge, as it can cause serious injury. Instead, flex and tighten the muscles being stretched. This will give you a safer more effective stretch. Breathe while holding your stretch rather than holding your breath.
- Incorporate stretching before working out, during a workout between sets, or afterward.
- Don't reserve stretching just for pre- and post-exercise. Take a half-hour a week and stretch your whole body. It's a great activity for while you're sitting in front of the TV. In just 30 minutes a week you'll have your dream body! Just kidding. You'll definitely feel better, though.
- Bob Anderson's book Stretching is considered the leading reference on the topic. This book should be in everyone's fitness library.
- There are also joint mobility exercises that can work your joints through their entire range of motion without necessarily stretching surrounding muscles. These exercises or movements generally use a back-and-forth or circular motion to improve joint mobility. They should always be done slowly with controlled motion to

avoid pushing a joint past its limits, since jerking or bouncing can cause injury to the joint.

Not only did we hold off putting this chapter in the book until the end, but we also didn't give it much space. This just does not seem to do stretching and flexibility justice! Stretching is simple but EXTREMELY IMPORTANT! Take the time to do it and reap the benefits.

Measuring Flexibility

How do you know if you need to improve your flexibility? Your trainer may check your flexibility with two simple tests. The **Sit and Reach** test measures the flexibility of the lower back and the backs of your legs. There is also an **Arm and Shoulder Stretch** which measures the flexibility of your shoulders and upper back. Lack of flexibility in these muscle groups usually indicates a need for overall improvement. When doing these "tests" don't jerk, bounce or force yourself to move further than is comfortable. To be safe, use slow, gentle movements when trying these tests. Your trainer will instruct you on how to do it properly.

No Time Like the Present

Stretching exercises can be done just about anywhere, anytime, and with very little interruption of your everyday routine. Stretching throughout the day relieves muscle tension and restores flexibility. These moments of stretching while you work will add up, and just a few minutes a day will help limber and warm up your muscles by aiding the circulation of oxygen-rich blood to them.

Simple Stretches

Here are some simple stretching exercises you can do at home. In each case, hold the stretch for about 10 seconds, relax, and then repeat the stretches 4 or 5 times. If a stretch hurts, relax it a little, or don't do it at all. Remember to always stretch slowly and smoothly, with no jerking or bouncing, which can cause injury. And keep breathing! For the following stretches, start by standing with your feet shoulder-width apart, knees relaxed, buttocks tucked under. Make sure your ears, shoulders, hips and ankles are in alignment.

- **Calf stretch**. Stand with one foot as far in front of the other as possible but while keeping both feet flat on the floor. Bending the front knee, slowly lean forward, keeping your rear heel pressed to the floor. (You may find it easier to do this against a wall or holding on to a chair.) Inhale and lift the rear heel off the floor, then, as you exhale, press the heel back onto the floor. Switch leg positions and repeat the pattern.
- **Quadriceps (front of the thigh) stretch**. Stand next to a chair and hold onto it with one hand for balance. Keeping one leg straight, bend the knee of the other behind you until you can grab your ankle with your free hand. Keep the bent leg parallel to the standing leg, and stretch gently backwards. You should feel the stretch in the front of the thigh.

For the following stretches, sit comfortably on the floor, with your arms hanging loosely by your sides. Arrange your torso so that your ears, shoulders, and hips are in line.

- **Head and neck roll**. Inhale, and as you exhale, let your head slowly roll forward until your chin is resting on your chest. Return to the starting position. Begin inhaling and slowly lower your right ear toward your right shoulder. (Don't lift the shoulder to meet your ear; keep it pressed down.) Continue to inhale as you slowly rotate your head past the shoulder and allow it to drop backwards. Let your mouth fall open. Now begin exhaling and rotate your head so your left ear is over your left shoulder. Still exhaling, slowly bring your head back to the starting position. Repeat this stretch a few times in each direction.

- **Shoulder rolls.** Press your shoulders forward, and raise them toward your ears. Then press the shoulders back as far as you can. Now lower them to the starting position. Each shoulder makes a complete circle. Repeat two or three times, then reverse direction. If you wish, you can rotate one shoulder at a time.
- **Arm stretch**. Raise your arms over your head. Interlace your fingers with palms facing up. Stretch your arms toward the ceiling.
- **Chest and back stretch.** Clasp your hands behind your head. Slowly push your elbows back as far as is comfortable.
- **Hamstring stretch**. Sit with one leg out and one leg bent so that the foot touches the upper thigh of the extended leg. Inhale as you sit up straight, then as you exhale, lean forward from the hips and grab the ankle of the straight leg. Repeat on each side. (A useful variation of this exercise is to pull with both hands on a belt or towel around your outstretched foot.)

For the following stretches, lie on the floor as indicated.

- **Lower back stretch**. Lie on your back with your hands behind your head and knees bent. Lift your feet off the floor, and bring your knees into your chest. Inhale and press your lower back into the floor. As you exhale, lift your head and shoulders off the floor and touch your forehead to your knees. Slowly lower your shoulders and head. Repeat several times.

- **Lower back stretch #2**. Roll over on your stomach. Place your palms on the floor beneath your shoulders, fingers forward. Keep your elbows close to your body. Inhale, stretch your chin forward, and slowly raise your head, neck, and chest off the floor. Keep your pelvis pressed to the floor. Exhale and slowly lower yourself

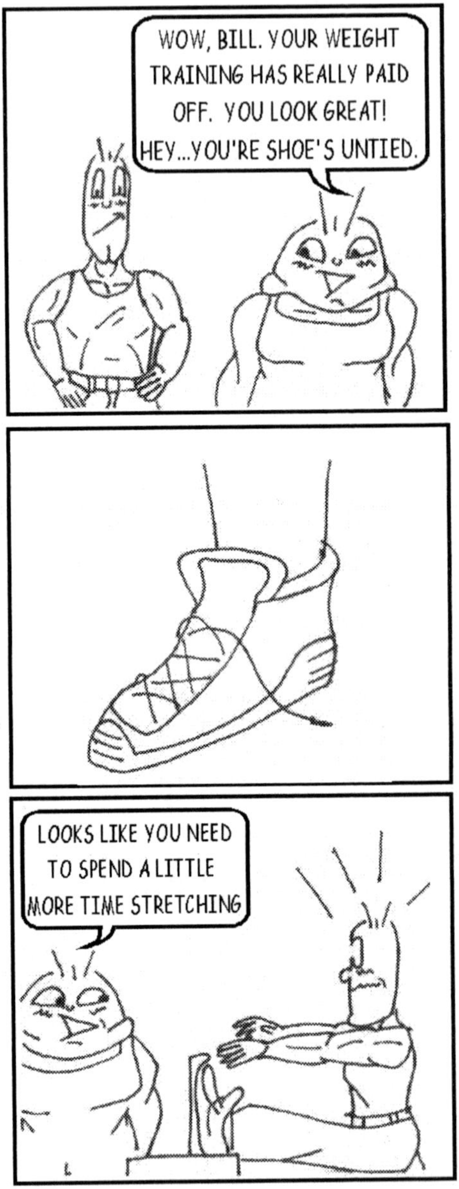

Summary – Chapter Nine

- Don't forget to stretch! Warm-up your muscles first and don't bounce.

Epilogue

What does a mechanical engineer know about nutrition and exercise?

Fair question.

You expect books on nutrition to be written by registered dietitians, and medical doctors. You would expect books on exercise to be written by exercise physiologists, PhD's, personal trainers, etc. In fact, there are many books available from these sources. You can find hundreds of books written by various experts in the field that tell you how you can lose weight, reduce your stress, feel better and/or get fit. These are the people that are highly trained in how the body works and what it takes to perform optimally. Right?

One thing that I have observed over the years is that many of the experts that write books or endorse products for nutrition and exercise have different approaches. As a result, there are conflicting opinions on what works and what doesn't. It seems to me that if all of these experts were taught at the same accredited universities, their teachings would be similar. In my engineering studies at UC Davis, our accredited program taught the same concepts of science and math as any other accredited engineering school. Newton's Laws of Motion were not taught as being open for interpretation. They work one way and one way only. The information flowing from the experts on nutrition should therefore be consistent, as they were all taught the same anatomy and physiology.

So why don't all the experts agree on the best method to be fit and healthy? Well, from what I can see, it has to do with money.

Fitness and weight loss is a multibillion dollar industry. 60

million Americans are obese and looking for a cure. This is a huge market that has spawned the creation of a huge weight loss industry. There is little question about it; there is a lot of money to be made in helping people get fit.

This is particularly true in the area of weight loss. Many "experts" have gained notoriety through their "unique" method of how to lose weight. This is a marketing ploy referred to as "differentiation". If you want to sell something, it is necessary to differentiate your product from the rest. For weight loss, the quicker the system helps drop the pounds, the better. Speed first, with safety being secondary. Look how many diet plan fads we have gone in the past 10 years. Come up with a hot new concept on how to lose weight and you can become rich. This is attractive to anyone that is in a health related field. The more new and different the concept is, the more likely you are to find a niche market for the concept. This lure of getting rich on American's #1 health concern has led many experts down a path of promoting different and potentially dangerous programs.

So where does that that leave us?

Confused.

We have all these experts telling us all these different things, and as a result we don't know what the truth of the matter is. We are stuck in a quagmire of distorted data and misapplied solutions. Help!

In all this mess, how do we find the truth? Not all the experts are wrong, but how do we find out which ones are right? How can we sort through all the studies and statistics to find out what the truth really is?

Engineers bridge the gap between pure science and the practical application of scientific principles. We are considered problem solvers, as we are trained to apply the data available from research to solve problems. For us, the best solution to a problem is the one that suits all the parameters the best. For example, for a given product, the best solutions might consider durability, safety, and expense.

The "best" fitness program should meet the following parameters:

1. *Long lasting results*. Any program which does not offer long-term results is not successful.
2. *Safety*. Long and short-term side effects must be considered.
3. *Improve how the participant feels*. Any plan that does not make the participant feel better is a failure. If you don't feel better, what's the point of the whole thing? Looking better is not enough.
4. *Reduce health risk for disease.*

These are some simple parameters for a successful fitness plan. Notice the parameters that were <u>not</u> listed:

- Weight loss. Losing weight is not an end in itself.
- Speed. How fast we get fit is not a criteria for a successful plan. My observation has been the faster one gets fit, the faster they get out of shape. Small, steady changes that last are what count.
- Easy to follow. We want to shed a light on fitness, but there is no easy fix to the problem. This has been the main issue with some of the programs from the "experts". They want to sell you an easy plan to lose weight. "Just take this pill" or "only 10 minutes per day". The light we shine will be on the truth of the matter, not on what you want to hear.

With the proper objective in mind, we explained what it takes to get and stay fit. We used the data and programs of many credible experts in the field and built an argument for what works. I also used my experience as a small club owner for the past 16 years to guide our research.

Many may still question why an engineer feels he can publish a book on the topic of nutrition and exercise. Others, however, will agree that it's about time an engineer got involved.

Ron Fay, P.E

Appendix 1

Credible Sources of Information

There are many credible sources for information and the majority of these sources agree on many of the key elements of health and fitness. A partial list of these sources are below.

We encourage you to research these sources. Take the time on the Internet or go to the library and read the books. The information is useful in that it will give you a more complete understanding of how your body works.

What's interesting about the sources is that, though their information is similar, the people or group's advocating the programs are very different. Some are medical doctors and dietitians, while others are government agencies. Others are personal trainers, who have proven the techniques and principles on others. This wide variety of sources only lends more credibility to the information.

Books

Transform
Author: Phil Kaplan
Overall program for fitness and nutrition.

Body for Life
Author: Bill Phillips
Overall program for fitness and nutrition.

Author: Miriam Nelson, Ph.D. (4 titles)

- **Strong Women, Strong Bones**
- **Strong Women Stay Young**
- **Strong Women Stay Slim**
- **Strong Women Eat Well**

Weight Training for Dummies
Liz Neporent, Suzanne Schlosberg

Eating Well for Optimum Health
Dr. Andrew Weil

Stretching
Bob Anderson

Sculpting Her Body Perfect
Brad Schoenfield

Websites

American College of Sports Medicine (ACSM) www.acsm.org

Centers for Disease Control and Prevention (CDC) www.cdc.gov

Department of Health and Human Services (HHS) www.hhs.gov

Office of the Surgeon General
www.surgeongeneral.gov

American Diabetes Association (ADA)
www.diabetes.org

American Dietetic Association
www.eatright.org

American Heart Association (AHA)
www.americanheart.org

American Cancer Society (ACS)
www.cancer.org

NYS Quit Line 866-697-8487 (866-NYQUITS) (smoking)
www.nysmokefree.com

Appendix 2

Nutritional Information

The following pages list some of the common foods we eat every day and the nutritional facts for these foods. For packaged products, check the "Nutrition Facts" labels for this information. For a more detailed list of foods and their nutritional values, see www.nutri-facts.com.

Vegetables

	Serving	Calories	Fat	Carbs	Dietary Fiber	Sugar	Protein
Asparagus	8 spears	25	0	4	2	2	2
Bell Pepper	1 med	30	0	7	2	4	1
Broccoli	1 med stalk	45	0.05	8	5	3	5
Cabbage	1 cup (cooked)	30	0	6.2	4.1	3.7	1.6
Carrot	7" long	35	0	8	2	5	1
Catsup	1 tbsp	16	0.1	4.1		3.9	0.2
Cauliflower	1/6 head	25	0	5	2	2	2
Celery	2 med	20	0	5	2	0	1
Cucumber	1/3 med	15	0	3	1	2	1
Green Beans	3/4 cup	25	0	5	3	2	1
Green Cabbage	1/12 med head	25	0	5	2	3	1
Green Onion	1/4 cup	10	0	2	1	1	0

	Serving	Calories	Fat	Carbs	Dietary Fiber	Sugar	Protein
Iceberg Lettuce	1/6 med	15	0	3	1	2	1
Leaf Lettuce	1.5 cups	15	0	4	2	2	1
Mushrooms	5 med	20	0	3	1	0	3
Onion	1 med	60	0	14	3	9	2
Peas	1/2 cup (cooked)	59	0.2	13	4.4	8.1	4.3
Potato	1 med	100	0	26	3	3	4
Radishes	7	15	0	3	0	2	1
Salsa	1/2 cup	32	0.8	1.5	0.1	1.4	0.4
Sauerkraut	1 cup (cooked)	27	0.2	6.1	3.6	2.5	1.3
Spinach	1 cup (cooked)	44.5	0.9	6.8	5.1	1.7	4.9
Summer Squash	1/2 med	20	0	4	2	2	1
Sweet Corn	1 med	80	1	18	3	5	3
Sweet Potato	1 med	130	0	33	4	7	2
Tomato	1 med	35	0.5	7	1	4	1
Tomato Juice	1 cup	41	0.1	10	1.9	8.4	1.8

Fruits

Apple	1 med	80	0	22	5	16	0
Apple Juice	1/2 cup	58	0.1	13.8	0.2	29	0.2
Apple Sauce	1/2 cup	53	0	13.8	1.5	15	0.4
Avocado	1/5	55	5	3	3	0	1
Banana	1 med	110	0	29	4	21	1

Fruits (cont'd)

	Serving	Calories	Fat	Carbs	Dietary Fiber	Sugar	Protein
Cantaloupe	1/4 med	50	0	12	1	11	1
Grape Juice	1 cup	154	0.2	37.8	0.3	37.5	1.4
Grapefruit	1/2 med	60	0	16	6	10	1
Grapes	1.5 cups	90	1	24	1	23	1
Honeydew	1/10 med	50	0	13	1	12	1
Kiwi	2 med	100	1	24	4	16	2
Lemon	1 med	15	0	5	1	1	0
Lime	1 med	20	0	7	2	0	0
Nectarine	1 med	70	0.5	16	2	12	1
Orange	1 med	70	0	21	7	14	1
Orange Juice	1 cup	112	0.5	25.8	0.5	25.3	1.7
Peach	1 med	40	0	10	2	9	1
Pear	1 med	100	1	25	4	17	1
Pineapple	2 slices	60	0	16	1	13	1
Plums	2 med	80	1	19	2	10	1
Raisins	1 oz.	84	0.2	23	1.2	21	0.7
Strawberries	8 med	45	0	12	4	8	1
Sweet Cherries	21 / 1 cup	90	0.5	22	3	19	2
Tangerine	1 med	50	0.5	15	3	12	1
Watermelon	2 cups	80	0	27	2	25	1

Starches (Breads and Cereals)

	Serving	Calories	Fat	Carbs	Dietary Fiber	Sugar	Protein
Pancakes	4"	86.3	3.5	11	0	11	2.6
Bagel, Small (27 g)	1 (2-1/2")	72	0.4	13.9	0.6	13.3	2.7
Bagel, Large (89 g)	1 (4")	245	1.4	47.5	2	45.5	9.3
Baked Beans	1 cup	236	1.1	52.1	12.7	39.4	12.2
Corn on the Cob	1 ear	83.2	1	19.3	2.2	17.1	2.6
Macaroni, cooked	1 cup	197	0.9	39.7	1.8	37.9	6.7
English Muffin	1 muffin	134	1	26.2	1.5	24.7	4.4
Egg Noodles	1 cup	213	2.4	40	1.8	38	7.6
Pasta, white, cooked	2 oz.	75	0.6	14.2	0	14.2	2.9
Potato, Baked	1 whole	220	0.2	51	4.8	46.2	4.6
Pretzels	10 twists	229	2.1	47.5	1.9	45.6	5.5
Rice Cakes	2 cakes	70	0.5	14.7	0.8	13.9	1.5
Rice	1 cup (cooked)	205	0.4	44.5	0.6	43.9	4.3
Toast, Whole Wheat	1 slice	65	1	11.8	1.2	10.6	2.3
Tortilla, Flour	1 pc	150	3.1	25.3	0	25.3	4.4

Proteins (Beans, Fish and Meat)

	Serving	Calories	Fat	Carbs	Dietary Fiber	Sugar	Protein
Abalone	3 oz.	90	0.6	5.1	0	5.1	14.5
Beans, baked	1 cup	236	1.1	52.1	12.7	39.4	12.2
Beans, Kidney	1 cup	207	0.8	38.1	9	29.1	13.3
Beans, Pinto	1 cup	206	1.9	36.6	11	25.6	11.7
Beef, Ground Round	3 oz.	218	13.9	0	0	0	21.6
Beef, Ground Lean	3 oz.	231	15.7	0	0	0	21
Chicken breast, Baked	1/2 breast (4 oz)	193	7.6	0	0	0	29.2
Chicken, dark meat	1 lb	256	15.9	0	0	0	26.2
Egg	1 large	78	5.3	0.6	0	0	6.3
Egg white	1 large white	17	0	0.3	0	0.3	3.5
Haddock	3 oz.	99	0.8	0	0	0	21.4
Halibut	3 oz.	119	2.5	0	0	0	22.7
Ham, sliced	1 oz (slice)	52	3	0.9	0	0.9	5
Peanut Butter	2 tbsp	190	16.3	6.2	1.9	4.3	8.1
Oysters	3 oz.	61.2	1.6	4.1	0	4.1	7
Perch	3 oz.	99.4	1	0	0	0	21.1
Salmon	3 oz.	99	2.9	0	0	0	16.9
Shrimp	3 oz.(16 large)	84.2	0.9	0	0	0	17.8
Tuna, water packed	3 oz	109	2.5	0	0	0	20
Turkey breast	4 oz	212	8.3	0	0	0	32.2

Dairy

	Serving	Calories	Fat	Carbs	Dietary Fiber	Sugar	Protein
Cheese, Cheddar	1 oz.	114	9.4	0.4	0	0.4	7.1
Cheese, Monterey	1 oz.	106	8.6	0.2	0	0.2	6.9
Cheese, Mozzarella	1 oz.	80	6.1	0.6	0	0.6	5.5
Cottage Cheese	4 oz.	117	5.1	3	0	3	14.1
Cottage Cheese, 2%	4 oz.	101	2.2	4.1	0	4.1	15.5
Milk	1 cup	150	8.1	11.4	0	11.4	8
Milk, 2%	1 cup	121	4.7	11.7	0	11.7	8.1
Milk, 1%	1 cup	102	2.6	11.7	0	11.7	8
Milk, Skim (0%)	1 cup	86	0.4	11.9	0	11.9	8.4
Yogurt, plain,skim	1 cup	137	0.4	18.8	0	18.8	14
Yogurt, frozen, lowfat	1/2 cup	115	4	17.4	0	17.4	2.9
Yogurt w/fruit	1 cup	250	2.6	46.7	0	46.7	11

Fats

	Serving	Calories	Fat	Carbs	Dietary Fiber	Sugar	Protein
Margarine or butter	1 tsp	34	3.8	0	0	0	0
Mayonnaise	1 tbsp	57	4.9	3.5	0	3.5	0.1
Mayonnaise, light	1 tbsp	50	4.9	1.3	0	1.3	0.1
Vegetable Oil	1 tbsp	124	14	0	0	0	0
Cream Cheese	1 tbsp	99	9.9	0.8	0	0.8	2.1
Cream Cheese, lite	1 oz	70	6	0	0	0	3
Sour Cream	1 tbsp	26	2.5	0.5	0	0.5	0.4
Sour Cream, lite	1 tbsp	20	1.8	0.6	0	0.6	0.4
Peanuts	1 oz.	160	13	6	2	1	7
Coffee Creamer	1 tbsp	20	1.7	0.6	0	0.6	0.4
Sunflower Seeds	1 oz.	165	14.1	6.8	2.6	4.2	5.5